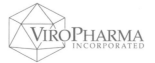

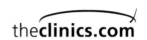
theclinics.com

IMMUNOLOGY AND ALLERGY CLINICS OF NORTH AMERICA

Angioedema

GUEST EDITOR
Bruce L. Zuraw, MD

CONSULTING EDITOR
Rafeul Alam, MD, PhD

November 2006 • Volume 26 • Number 4

SAUNDERS

An Imprint of Elsevier, Inc.
PHILADELPHIA   LONDON   TORONTO   MONTREAL   SYDNEY   TOKYO

W.B. SAUNDERS COMPANY
A Division of Elsevier Inc.

Elsevier, Inc., 1600 John F. Kennedy Blvd., Suite 1800, Philadelphia, PA 19103-2899

http://www.theclinics.com

IMMUNOLOGY AND ALLERGY CLINICS   Volume 26, Number 4
OF NORTH AMERICA   ISSN 0889-8561
November 2006   ISBN 1-4160-3809-4
Editor: Carla Holloway   978-1-4160-3809-2

The ideas and opinions expressed in *Immunology and Allergy Clinics of North America* do not necessarily reflect those of the Publisher. The Publisher does not assume any responsibility for any injury and/or damage to persons or property arising out of or related to any use of the material contained in this periodical. The reader is advised to check the appropriate medical literature and the product information currently provided by the manufacturer of each drug to be administered to verify the dosage, the method and duration of administration, or contraindications. It is the responsibility of the treating physician or other health care professional, relying on independent experience and knowledge of the patient, to determine drug dosages and the best treatment for the patient. Mention of any product in this issue should not be construed as endorsement by the contributors, editors, or the Publisher of the product or manufacturers' claims.

Immunology and Allergy Clinics of North America (ISSN 0889-8561) is published quarterly by Elsevier Inc., 360 Park Avenue South, New York, NY 10010-1710. Months of issue are February, May, August, and November. Business and Editorial offices: 1600 John F. Kennedy Blvd., Suite 1800, Philadelphia, PA 19103-2899. Customer Service office: 6277 Sea Harbor Drive, Orlando, FL 32887-4800. Periodicals postage paid at New York, NY and additional mailing offices. Subscription prices are $215.00 per year for US individuals, $308.00 per year for US institutions, $215.00 per year for US students and residents, $215.00 per year for Canadian individuals, and students, $374.00 per year for Canadian institutions, $253.00 per year for international individuals, $374.00 per year for international institutions, $248.00 per year for international students. To receive student/resident rate, orders must be accompanied by name of affiliated institution, date of term, and the *signature* of program/residency coordinator on institution letterhead. Orders will be billed at individual rate until proof of status is received. Foreign air speed delivery is included in all *Clinics* subscription prices. All prices are subject to change without notice. POSTMASTER: Send address changes to *Immunology and Allergy Clinics of North America*, Elsevier Periodicals Customer Service, 6277 Sea Harbor Drive, Orlando, FL 32887-4800. **Customer Service: 1-800-654-2452 (US). From outside of the US, call 1-407-345-4000. E-mail: hhspcs@wbsaunders.com**.

Reprints. For copies of 100 or more, of articles in this publication, please contact the Commercial Reprints Department, Elsevier Inc., 360 Park Avenue South, New York, New York 10010-1710. Tel. (212) 633-3813 Fax: (212) 462-1935 e-mail: reprints@elsevier.com.

Immunology and Allergy Clinics of North America is covered in Index Medicus, Current Contents/Life Sciences, Science Citation Index, ISI/BIOMED, Chemical Abstracts, and EMBASE/Excerpta Medica.

Printed in the United States of America.

CONSULTING EDITOR

RAFEUL ALAM, MD, PhD, Veda and Chauncey Ritter Chair in Immunology; Professor and Director, Division of Allergy and Immunology, National Jewish Medical and Research Center, University of Colorado at Denver Health Sciences Center, Denver, Colorado

GUEST EDITOR

BRUCE L. ZURAW, MD, Professor of Medicine, Veteran's Administration Medical Center, University of California San Diego, La Jolla, California

CONTRIBUTORS

ALBERT ADAM, PhD, Professor, Faculty of Pharmacy, University of Montreal, Montréal, Quebec, Canada

ALEENA BANERJI, MD, Division of Rheumatology, Allergy and Immunology, Massachusetts General Hospital, Harvard Medical School, Boston, Massachusetts

KONRAD BORK, MD, Professor, Department of Dermatology, Johannes Gutenberg University, Mainz, Germany

NANCY J. BROWN, MD, Robert H. Williams Professor of Medicine and Professor of Pharmacology, Division of Clinical Pharmacology, Vanderbilt University School of Medicine, Nashville, Tennessee

JAMES BRIAN BYRD, MD, Research Fellow in Medicine, Division of Clinical Pharmacology, Vanderbilt University School of Medicine, Nashville, Tennessee

ROBERTO CASTELLI, MD, Department of Internal Medicine, IRCCS Fondazione Ospedale Maggiore Policlinico, Milan, Italy

LORENZA CHIARA ZINGALE, MD, Department of Internal Medicine, San Giuseppe Hospital—AFaR, University of Milan, Milan, Italy

MARCO CICARDI, MD, Professor, Department of Internal Medicine, San Giuseppe Hospital—AFaR, University of Milan, Milan, Italy

ALVIN E. DAVIS III, MD, Professor of Pediatrics, CBR Institute for Biomedical Research, Harvard Medical School, Boston, Massachusetts

MICHAEL M. FRANK, MD, Samuel L. Katz Professor of Pediatrics, Medicine, and Immunology, Duke University Medical Center, Durham, North Carolina

EVANGELO FRIGAS, MD, Consultant, Division of Allergic Diseases and Internal Medicine; and Associate Professor of Medicine, Mayo Clinic College of Medicine, Rochester, Minnesota

PAUL A. GREENBERGER, MD, Division of Allergy-Immunology, Department of Medicine, Northwestern University, Feinberg School of Medicine, Chicago, Illinois

C. ERIK HACK, MD, PhD, Crucell Nederland NV, Leiden, the Netherlands; Department of Clinical Chemistry, VU Medical Center, Amsterdam, the Netherlands

MIGUEL PARK, MD, Senior Associate Consultant, Division of Allergic Diseases and Internal Medicine; and Instructor of Medicine, Mayo Clinic College of Medicine, Rochester, Minnesota

JAVID SHEIKH, MD, Division of Allergy and Inflammation, Beth Israel Deaconess Medical Center, Harvard Medical School, Boston, Massachusetts

INEKE G.A. WAGENAAR-BOS, PhD, Department of Immunopathology, Sanquin Research at CLB, Landsteiner Laboratory, Academical Medical Center, University of Amsterdam, Amsterdam, the Netherlands

DAVID WELDON, MD, Assistant Professor of Internal Medicine, Texas A & M University Health Sciences Center, College Station, Texas

PETER F. WELLER, MD, Divisions of Allergy and Inflammation and Infectious Diseases, Beth Israel Deaconess Medical Center, Harvard Medical School, Boston, Massachusetts

ANDREA ZANICHELLI, MD, Department of Internal Medicine, San Giuseppe Hospital—AFaR, University of Milan, Milan, Italy

BRUCE L. ZURAW, MD, Professor of Medicine, Veteran's Administration Medical Center, University of California San Diego, La Jolla, California

CONTENTS

> Angioedema is a swelling of a defined area that typically lasts for
> no longer than a few days. However, allergists will often be con-
> sulted on cutaneous reactions that do not (by history) suggest an-
> gioedema nor appear to be consistent with angioedema. Most of
> the conditions that present with swelling are due to dependent
> edema, infections, or medication side effects. However, angio-
> edema can be a result of autoimmune conditions that present with
> angioedema and not urticaria. A high index of suspicion for other
> conditions should help in the differential diagnoses.

> Heterozygous deficiency of C1-inhibitor (C1-INH) leads to the clin-
> ical picture of hereditary angioedema (HAE). C1-INH is a serine
> protease inhibitor (serpin). C1-INH is unique among serpins in that
> it has a unique N-terminal domain, which has no homology with
> any known protein, in addition to its serpin domain. In this article
> the authors summarize current insights into the biochemical me-
> chanism of serpins in general and discuss the structure and func-
> tion of C1-INH in light of these insights. In addition, structural
> consequences of mutations in C1-INH as occurring in patients
> who have HAE are discussed. Finally, the possible functions of
> the unique N-terminal domain are reviewed.

Mechanism of Angioedema in First Complement Component Inhibitor Deficiency

Alvin E. Davis III

Since shortly after the discovery that hereditary angioedema resulted from deficiency of first complement component (C1) inhibitor, the characterization of the mediator of angioedema has been a major goal. However, because C1 inhibitor regulates activation of both the contact and complement systems, identification of the mediator was not immediately accomplished. For a number of years, some studies appeared to indicate involvement of one system, whereas other studies suggested involvement of the other. However, the vast majority of the evidence accumulated over the past several years indicates quite clearly that the major mediator is bradykinin. Therefore, unregulated contact system activation is the defect that leads directly to the development of angioedema.

Hereditary Angioedema: The Clinical Syndrome and its Management in the United States

Michael M. Frank

There have been important breakthroughs in the understanding and treatment of hereditary anigoedema (HAE). An associated abnormality of the serum protein C1 inhibitor led to purified protein use to end attacks. Consideration of endocrine functions led to rediscovery of impeded androgen use in disease prophylaxis. Considerations of pathophysiology led to introduction of epsilon aminocaproic and tranexemic acids in prophylaxis and to a resurgence in trials of new therapeutic agents. We have gone from a situation where it was not uncommon for patients to have a severe attack sometime in their lives that led to airway compromise and possible death to a situation where death from disease is highly unusual. Thus HAE is in many ways a success story of modern medicine.

Acquired Deficiency of the Inhibitor of the First Complement Component: Presentation, Diagnosis, Course, and Conventional Management

Lorenza Chiara Zingale, Roberto Castelli, Andrea Zanichelli, and Marco Cicardi

Acquired deficiency of the inhibitor of the first complement component (C1-INH) is a rare, potentially life-threatening disease whose cause, course, and management are not completely defined. This article analyzes the etiopathogenetic mechanism, the clinical presentation, and the relationship between acquired C1-INH deficiency and lymphoproliferative disorders. Moreover, the authors give an overview of the outcome of the disease and the different therapies proposed to cure it.

FORTHCOMING ISSUES

RECENT ISSUES

VISIT THESE RELATED WEB SITES

Access your subscription at:
www.theclinics.com

ELSEVIER
SAUNDERS

Immunol Allergy Clin N Am
26 (2006) xi–xii

IMMUNOLOGY
AND ALLERGY
CLINICS
OF NORTH AMERICA

Foreword

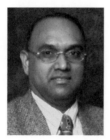

Rafeul Alam, MD, PhD
Consulting Editor

Angioedema, especially laryngeal angioedema, is one of the most dreadful conditions in medicine. Angioedema can be as dramatic as anaphylaxis and other life-threatening conditions in its clinical presentation. However, there is an important difference between angioedema and anaphyalxis. The latter, if intervened early, could be effectively treated in health care facilities. The same is not true for angioedema. Despite the progress in medicine in so many areas we still do not have any rapidly active treatment for laryngeal edema other than intubation, fresh frozen plasma and supportive care.

For more than 40 years, C1 esterase deficiency (absolute or relative) has been considered the cause of many forms of angioedema. How this deficiency causes plasma leakage through the endothelium and swelling of the soft tissue remains a mystery. The finding that first-generation ACE inhibitors cause angioedema in some patients independent of complement pointed to the existence of multiple mechanisms for angioedema formation. There are a number of new developments in this seemingly stagnant area. First, the mechanism of edema formation is becoming better understood and the nature of the mediators is better defined. Especially, the involvement of bradykinin and kinin-generating system in angioedema formation is better appreciated. Second, clinical trials with several new therapeutic agents have been completed or ongoing, giving hope for effective therapeutic interventions. More importantly, there is hope for treatment of acute laryngeal and visceral angioedema with C1 esterase concentrate preparations. Finally,

doi:10.1016/j.iac.2006.10.001

new subtypes of angioedema (estrogen-dependent and independent) have been identified in which C1 esterase activity and C4 level are normal.

These exciting developments prompted us to revisit this rare but important disease. Dr. Bruce Zuraw, an internationally renowned expert in the field, has invited a distinguished group of scientists and clinical investigators to update us on the pathogenesis and treatment of angioedema. The future looks quite hopeful.

Rafeul Alam, MD, PhD
Division of Immunology and Allergy
National Jewish Medical and Research Center
University of Colorado at Denver Health Sciences Center
1400 Jackson Street
Denver, CO 80206, USA

E-mail address: alamr@njc.org

ELSEVIER
SAUNDERS

Immunol Allergy Clin N Am
26 (2006) xiii–xv

IMMUNOLOGY
AND ALLERGY
CLINICS
OF NORTH AMERICA

Preface

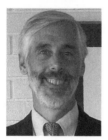

Bruce L. Zuraw, MD
Guest Editor

I was surprised and pleased to learn that the *Immunology and Allergy Clinics of North America* would devote an entire issue to angioedema. Remarkable progress has been made in unraveling the pathogenesis of angioedema, leading to important advances in treatment modalities. These developments have galvanized the interest of affected patients and treating physicians. This issue reviews the spectrum of angioedema to provide a framework for approaching the management of these patients.

Angioedema occurs both in conjunction with or separately from the more common swelling disorder, urticaria. A variety of other conditions can mimic some aspects of angioedema, and clinicians must be aware of the spectrum of swelling disorders that can be confused with true angioedema. Establishing the correct diagnosis is a critical step in selecting the appropriate management plan. The first article in this issue reviews the differential diagnosis of angioedema, focusing on disorders that can masquerade as angioedema.

The next seven articles address types of angioedema that classically occur in the absence of urticaria. Such a presentation suggests several potential diagnoses, specifically hereditary angioedema, acquired angioedema, or angioedema associated with angiotensin-converting enzyme inhibitors or angiotensin receptor blockers. Since Virginia Donaldson identified the cause of hereditary angioedema as a deficiency of C1 inhibitor in 1963, the biology of C1 inhibitor has been a topic of considerable interest. The second article in this issue reviews our current understanding of the structure and function of C1 inhibitor and the impact of different C1 inhibitor mutations, while the third article summarizes how the development of C1 inhibitor knockout mice along with careful evaluation of patients with hereditary angioedema have provided convincing evidence that bradykinin is the major mediator of swelling in hereditary angioedema. The fourth and fifth articles then review the clinical spectrum of hereditary and acquired C1 inhibitor deficiency, including clinical presentation, diagnosis, and management. Although considered an orphan disease, hereditary angioedema is currently the focus of five ongoing or recently completed clinical studies involving four different types of agents. The sixth article reviews these new agents and discusses how they may alter the treatment patterns of hereditary angioedema patients.

In recent years, a novel hereditary form of angioedema has been described that is not related to C1 inhibitor deficiency, and which in some cases appears to be estrogen-dependent. The seventh article in this issue reviews what has been learned about type III hereditary angioedema, and discusses potential heterogeneity within this population. Angioedema related to angiotensin-converting enzyme inhibitors has become an increasingly important problem as the use of these drugs has increased, and is now a common cause of hospitalization. The eighth article reviews angioedema that is caused by exposure to angiotensin-converting enzyme inhibitor or, to a lesser degree, angiotensin receptor blockers.

The most common cause of recurrent angioedema is idiopathic, and continues to present the clinician with a daunting challenge in diagnosis and particularly in management. The ninth article in this issue reviews idiopathic recurrent angioedema and provides a structured model to approach the care of these patients. Angioedema can be mistaken for anaphylaxis and vice versa; furthermore, larygneal angioedema is one of the most severe manifestations of anaphylaxis. Angioedema in both anaphylactic and anaphylactoid reactions is reviewed in the tenth article. The final article then reviews the fascinating relationship between cytokines and angioedema that is seen in episodic angioedema with eosinophilia, nonepisodic angioedema, and angioedema associated with cytokine treatment.

This is an exciting time for patients with hereditary angioedema, as 40 years of research are about to be transformed into significant clinical advances that will have a substantial impact on the lives of affected patients. Realization of this goal, however, will require the medical community to improve our efforts to recognize and diagnose affected patients. Hopefully the articles in this issue will not only convey what has been learned about angioedema, but will also highlight areas where our understanding is incomplete or our treatment modalities remain unequal to the challenge.

Bruce L. Zuraw, MD
Veteran's Administration Medical Center
University of California San Diego
9500 Gilman Drive, Mail Code 0732
La Jolla, CA 92093, USA

E-mail address: bzuraw@ucsd.edu

ELSEVIER
SAUNDERS

Immunol Allergy Clin N Am
26 (2006) 603–613

IMMUNOLOGY
AND ALLERGY
CLINICS
OF NORTH AMERICA

Differential Diagnosis of Angioedema

David Weldon, MD

*Texas A&M University Health Sciences Center, 1600 University Drive East,
College Station, TX 77840, USA*

Angioedema is defined as transient swelling of defined areas in the deep dermis or subcutaneous tissue resulting from vascular leakage. Angioedematous lesions tend to be large, pale, nonpruritic (although they may be painful or burning), and occur anywhere on the body. While the duration of swelling in angioedema is sometimes short like urticaria (that often accompanies angioedema), the swelling of angioedema typically persists for a day or more and occasionally can last for multiple days before remitting.

A variety of other pathophysiologic processes may cause swelling that superficially resemble angioedema. Although the majority of these conditions do not respond to antihistamines or other medications used to treat urticaria and angioedema, they nonetheless may be mistakenly called "angioedema," and frequently are treated with parenteral or oral glucocorticoids. Because the management of these disorders is generally distinct from the management of angioedema, it is important to carefully distinguish angioedema from other causes of swelling. Based on the patient's recollection of the onset and duration of swelling together with key signs and symptoms, the astute clinician can generally distinguish angioedema from those conditions that resemble angioedema. This article will briefly review the major causes of angioedema, then discuss other non-angioedematous conditions that may masquerade as and be mistaken for angioedema.

Angioedema

Angioedema is a result of interstitial edema from mediators affecting capillary and venule permeability. The swelling due to angioedema involves tissues deeper than the dermis and thus appears and feels different than urticaria. Upwards of 50% of patients with urticaria may have angioedema concurrently [1]. The mechanisms responsible for the swelling in both

---

E-mail address: dweldon@swmail.sw.org

urticaria and angioedema are generally similar. A major exception to this, however, is the angioedema associated with C-1 esterase inhibitor deficiency, which is caused by a distinct pathophysiologic mechanism (see the article by Davis elsewhere in this issue) and is not accompanied by urticaria [2].

Several clinical clues help distinguish angioedema from other causes of swelling. In most instances, the involvement is in highly vascular areas (eg, lips, oropharynx, peri-orbital region). The region involved is not symmetric (eg, only one side of the face involved) and typically does not favor dependent areas. Angioedema is also transient, a given lesion typically lasting 24 to 48 hours then resolving. Unlike urticaria, the sensation associated with angioedema is more painful or burning than pruritic.

Allergic angioedema

An allergic (IgE-mediated) etiology is typically considered first when patients present for evaluation of acute angioedema. Possible allergic basis of the angioedema is often suggested by a careful history that uncovers a relationship between the onset of swelling and exposure to foods, stinging insects, latex, medications, or aeroallergens (as in the case of angioedema seen with allergic conjunctivitis). Cutaneous contact with some allergens has also been shown to cause angioedema. Angioedema frequently accompanies anaphylaxis, which is a systemic allergic reaction typically including hypotension, urticaria, or difficulty breathing.

Nonallergic angioedema

Chronic recurrent angioedema

Chronic recurrent idiopathic angioedema is most commonly seen in the presence of concomitant chronic idiopathic urticaria, but can also occur without urticaria (see the article by Frigas and Park elsewhere in this issue). In addition, some of the physical urticarias can be mistaken for angioedema. Depending on the surface area involved, patients with acquired cold-induced urticaria may have extensive involvement mimicking angioedema of an extremity. Patients with vibration-induced urticaria/angioedema have angioedema as the most likely presenting symptom [3]. Patients with vibratory angioedema may have swelling of their hands as their chief complaint. Delayed pressure urticaria typically presents with subcutaneous discomfort and swelling that is more consistent with angioedema than urticaria [4]. Typically patients complain of discomfort in areas of pressure (eg, beltline, backs of legs, feet) yet often this diagnosis is difficult to confirm even with a properly performed challenge.

Pharmaceuticals causing angioedema on a non-IgE–mediated basis

Some pharmaceutical agents may promote angioedema from non-IgE–mediated mechanisms. Angiotensin-converting enzyme (ACE) inhibitors can cause angioedema, presumably through their ability to interfere with the degradation of bradykinin (see the article by Byrd and colleagues elsewhere in this issue) [5]. Angioedema as a result of ACE inhibitors typically occurs shortly after starting the medication [6], although some cases have been reported to be delayed months after initiation of the medication [7]. Although there are rare reports of angioedema associated with angiotensin receptor blockers (ARB) [8], most patients with ACE inhibitor–induced angioedema are able to successfully switch to an ARB without recurrence of their angioedema [9]. Ionic radiocontrast material agents can promote anaphylactoid reactions including angioedema, presumably because of changes in serum osmolarity (see the article by Greenberger elsewhere in this issue) [10]. Aspirin and other nonsteroidal anti-inflammatory drugs (NSAIDs) can induce angioedema by their ability to inhibit cyclo-oxygenase 1 (COX-1) and thus presumably favoring cysteinyl leukotriene production [11]. Angioedema can be provoked in an estrogen-dependent manner in some individuals, and this appears to be transmitted in a hereditary manner (see the article by Bork elsewhere in this issue) [12].

Angioedema associated with eosinophilia

Hypereosinophilic syndrome (HES) is characterized by a blood eosinophilia of greater than $1500/\mu L$ for longer than 6 months, evidence of end-organ (cardiac, pulmonary, neurologic) dysfunction, and no other medical reason for the eosinophilia [13]. Angioedema or urticaria may occur with HES and patients are more likely to have a benign course if HES presents only with angioedema [14]. Patients presenting with weight gain (upwards of 18% of their total body weight), along with fever and marked peripheral eosinophilia with elevated IgM may have episodic angioedema with eosinophilia (Gleich's syndrome) (see the article by Banerji and colleagues elsewhere in this issue). This condition is differentiated from HES because of central organ involvement found in HES [15]. A nonepisodic version of angioedema with eosinophilia has been reported that is characterized by absence of recurrent attacks of angioedema, occurring in females, without an elevation in IgM. In contrast to Gleich's syndrome, the nonepisodic version affects the extremeties and has a more benign course [16].

Angioedema associated with C1 inhibitor deficiency

As mentioned above, C1 inhibitor deficiency is associated with recurrent angioedema not accompanied by urticaria. This can occur both on a hereditary basis (hereditary angioedema, see the article by Frank elsewhere in this issue) as well as on an acquired basis (see the article by Zingale and colleagues elsewhere in this issue).

Masqueraders of angioedema

The causes of angioedema discussed above are all well known to allergists and to most clinicians. However, other cutaneous reactions that mimic angioedema should be considered in the differential diagnoses. The majority of these reactions are rare but serve to demonstrate that not everything that causes swelling should be treated with antihistamines or corticosteroids. Box 1 lists many conditions that present with swelling that may be mistaken for angioedema.

Contact dermatitis

Patients with contact dermatitis due to exposure to antigens eliciting delayed-type hypersensitivity responses often present with angioedema of the face and periorbital region. Rhus dermatitis from contact with poison ivy is notorious for producing isolated swelling affecting one eye and especially in children. Although angioedema-like swelling may be the first manifestation of contact dermatitis, the reaction usually declares itself with the production of vesicles or blisters, and later an eczematous dermatitis that lasts for days to weeks.

Box 1. Conditions that mimic angioedema

Contact dermatitis
Rhus (Poison ivy, oak)
Trauma or burns
Acute idiopathic scrotal edema
Autoantibodies (hypocomplementemic urticarial vasculitis
  syndrome)
Weber-Christian disease
Tumor necrosis factor receptor–associated periodic syndrome
Thyroid orbitopathy
Well's syndrome
Schulman's syndrome
Blepharochalasis
Clarkson syndrome
Dependent edema
Marasmus, hypoproteinemia
Superior vena cava syndrome
Infections
Viral (Parvo, herpes)
Bacterial (cellulitis)
Parasite (Loa loa, Trichenella)
Scleromyxedema
Systemic amyloidosis
Melkersson-Rosenthal syndrome
Crohn's disease
Acquired C1-inhibitor deficiency syndrome

Dependent edema

Patients with underlying medical conditions that cause dependent edema may have areas that are misconstrued as angioedema. Most likely, edema that develops in the lower legs in an older patient with underlying heart disease would be appropriately ascribed to vascular insufficiency or underlying congestive heart failure. Decreased plasma oncotic pressure is also associated with edema. However, more persistent edema may be related to vascular malformations that may especially involve the lymphatic system. Acute exacerbations of chronic edema may develop blisters (stasis blisters or hydrostatic bullae) that can sometimes be confused with an immune-mediated reaction [17].

In some instances, the obstruction may be central with edema that becomes noticeable only when the patient is dependent. Superior vena cava obstruction due to tumors may present with edema when the patient is supine or prone, yet the edema gradually resolves when the patient is upright. Cough and dyspnea are usually associated with this and the patient usually has swelling involving the upper (but not the lower) extremities as well as the face and neck [18].

Trauma may result in angioedema. Burns (especially superficial sunburns) may be associated with mild angioedema. Quincke's disease may result from thermal injury as in the case of a patient who had inhaled cocaine smoke and developed marked swelling of his uvula [19]. Acute idiopathic scrotal edema in young boys occurs in children from ages 2 to 10 years of age. Patients present with painful unilateral scrotal swelling due to thickening of the scrotal sac but without hydrocele. Erythema also accompanies the swelling, with demarcation that may extend to the perineum, abdomen, or penis and mimics cellulitis. However, the patient is afebrile and the condition resolves within days without antibiotics [20].

Infections

Some infections may present with swelling that can be diagnosed as angioedema. Such infections persist until treated and thus must be differentiated from acute angioedema. Parasite infections can cause angioedema around the eyes. Romana's sign is unilateral angioedema of one eye that occurs with American trypanosimiasis. Trichinosis can also cause periorbital edema with peripheral eosinophilia. Tropical filariasis can cause lymphatic obstruction with resultant swelling of the affected limb or can cause swelling of the eyeball (*Loa loa*) [21].

Bacterial infections may also mimic angioedema. Cellulitis (especially facial) is associated with erythema, swelling, and fever and is usually differentiated from angioedema. Rosacea may also present with swelling of the face and be mistaken for angioedema of the eyes or cheeks. In some instances, acne vulgaris may be extensive and involve swelling of the area [21].

Viral infections are frequently associated with urticaria in children. Parvovirus B19 has been described as a cause of angioedema in neonates [22]. In some instances, edema may precede the appearance of herpes infections including herpetic zoster.

Vasculitis and panniculitis

Autoantibodies are also found commonly in systemic lupus erythematosis (SLE). This can promote both urticaria and angioedema due to consumption of complement from autoantibodies to the collagen-like fragment of C1q [23]. Hypocomplementemic urticarial vasculitis syndrome has also been noted to cause angioedema in patients with SLE. Although this condition responds to immunosuppressants, rarely are monoclonal antibodies such as rituximab required [24].

Weber-Christian disease is a panniculitis with fever and swelling that may mimic angioedema [25]. This condition is characterized by fever, subcutaneous nodules, and involvement of subcutaneous fat. Two patients have been described with panniculitis and a mutation of the tumor necrosis receptor super family known as tumor necrosis factor receptor–associated periodic syndrome (TRAPS). Both patients responded to etanercept [26].

Mucinoses and other infiltrating disorders

Perhaps the most commonly considered endocrinopathy associated with edema that simulates angioedema is autoimmune thyroid disease. Thyroid orbitopathy is a condition characterized by gradual swelling of the periorbital area. It is usually associated with hypothyroidism and resolves after treatment with thyroid hormone supplement. Graves' disease may also present with orbitopathy. Other edematous manifestations of thyroid disease include myxedema of the face with severe hypothyroidism and pretibial myxedema seen in Graves' disease. The latter is characterized by waxy indurated nodules or plaques that may have a *peau d'orange* appearance [27]. Both conditions are a result of the accumulation of mucin within the dermis. In pretibial myxedema, perivascular lymphocytic infiltrate with mast cells may be similar to the pathology of urticaria except that large stellate fibroblasts are also seen in addition to the mucin amidst collagen bundles [28].

Scleromyxedema can present with swelling of the forehead along with small, waxy papules. Long and deep longitudinal furrows across the forehead may give the patient a lionoid appearance. Induration of other areas (especially the forearm) may simulate swelling. Scleromyxedema is most often associated with a paraproteinemia (most often IgG with λ light chains) and in 10% of affected patients, progresses to multiple myeloma [29].

Macroglossia can be mistaken for angioedema of the tongue. Most often, macroglossia is associated with systemic amyloidosis. Dental impressions on the tongue that do not fade are a clue of the infiltration by AL protein in the area. Other signs such as periorbital ecchymoses and waxy, translucent facial papules may also be present. Primary systemic amyloidosis is usually associated with a plasma cell dyscrasia [30].

Eosinophilic dermatoses

Infiltrative disorders with eosinophils may present with large erythematous plaques or induration of subcutaneous tissue that may be mistaken for angioedema. Wells' syndrome presents as recurrent and often painful plaques that resemble cellulitis. Fever, peripheral eosinophilia, and malaise accompany the onset of the plaques. Biopsy reveals dense infiltration by eosinophils with characteristic flame figures from collagen fibers coated with eosinophil granules [31]. Shulman's syndrome (eosinophilic fasciitis) may present with edema, pain, and tenderness of the affected extremities. An elevated sedimentation rate, marked peripheral eosinophilia, elevated aldolase, and hyperglobulinemia are seen. Early diagnosis is important to prevent muscle contractures and loss of mobility [32]. A similar condition has been reported to occur with contaminants in tryptophan causing eosinophilic myalgia syndrome [33].

Orofacial swelling alone

Melkersson Rosenthal syndrome is a condition characterized by persistent swelling of the lips due to noncaseating granulomatous infiltration of the lips. It is typically associated with a fissured tongue (lingua plicata), orofacial edema, and facial nerve palsy. However, the classic triad is seen in a minority of cases [34]. Other areas of the face (eyelids, periorbital region) may present with persistent swelling as a variation of this syndrome [35]. Crohn's disease and sarcoidosis may also present with cheilits granulomatosa but without facial paralysis or fissured tongue [36,37]. Rarely, a contact dermatitis may mimic chelitis granulomatosa. Fig. 1 shows a young woman

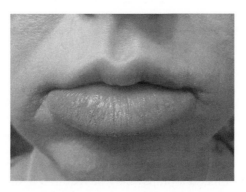

Fig. 1. Lower lip swelling in a patient simulating chelitis granulomatosa.

with Crohn's disease who had persistent angioedema of her lower lip that proved to be due to blistering delayed hypersensitivity to *Saccharomyces sp* after percutaneous testing.

Parotid gland involvement by sarcoidosis occurs in 6% of sarcoidosis patients and may cause swelling of the cheek confused with persistent angioedema. Likewise, a ranula is obstruction of a sublingual gland that may mimic angioedema [38].

Cheilitis glandularis is a rare condition that affects older men. It is characterized by hypertrophy of the lower lip that can mimic persistent (yet mild) angioedema and stinging of the lower lip. Close examination reveals secretory ducts that are inflamed with resultant red mucosal macules [39]. Scleredema adultorum of Buschke is a very rare infiltrative condition characterized by increased collagen and glycosaminolgycans that may present with persistent periorbital edema [40].

Blepharochalasis is a condition of the eyelids characterized by recurrent episodes of nonpruritic swelling that eventually causes visual field impairment and warrants surgical correction. Unlike festoons, which develop under the eyes, blepharochalasis involves both upper and lower eyelids [41].

Lymphoproliferative and autoimmune disorders

Acquired C1 inhibitor deficiency and angioedema (described earlier in this article) occurs as a consequence of lymphoproliferative disorders in some cases [42]. Clarkson syndrome from a capillary leak syndrome due to monoclonal gammopathy can precipitate angioedema and lymphedema [43].

In children, angioedema associated with a subsequent erythematopapular rash may be a presenting sign of autoimmune lymphoproliferative syndrome (ALPS) [44]. This entity is a result of a disorder in lymphocyte apoptosis involving the Fas-dependent pathway [45]. Facial edema precedes the onset of acute hemorrhagic edema, which is a leukocytoclastic vasculitis that is characterized by large annular or purpuric lesions on the extremities of a febrile child [46].

Dermatomyositis has been considered by some authors to be in the differential diagnosis of angioedema, possibly related to the poikiloderma of the face and the persistent edema of the eyelids [47].

Summary

There are many conditions that may present with swelling that mimics angioedema. When swelling persists for greater than a few days or is unresponsive to treatment for urticaria/angioedema, other etiologies should be considered. In most instances, a thorough history and physical examination will define other etiologies. However, for more persistent conditions, further laboratory evaluation and a biopsy may be required to define the diagnosis. Rarely is a more aggressive approach required to make the diagnosis.

Clinicians should remember that if the swelling does not act like angioedema, it more than likely is not angioedema.

References

[1] Champion RH, Roberts SOB, Carpenter RG, et al. Urticaria and angioedema. A review of 554 patients. Br J Dermatol 1969;81:588–92.

[2] Agostoni A, Aygoren-Pursun E, Binkley KE, et al. Hereditary and acquired angioedema: proceedings of the third C1 esterase inhibitor deficiency workshop and beyond. J Allergy Clin Immunol 2004;114:S51–131.

[3] Lawlor F, Black AK, Breathnach AS, et al. Vibratory angioedema: lesion induction, clinical features, laboratory and ultrastructural findings and response to therapy. Br J Dermatol 1989;120:93–9.

[4] Lawlor F, Black AK. Delayed pressure urticaria. Immunol Allergy Clin North Am 2004;24: 247–58.

[5] Anderson MW, deShazo RD. Studies of the mechanism of angiotensin-converting enzyme (ACE) inhibitor-associated angioedema: the effect of an ACE inhibitor on cutaneous responses to bradykinin, codeine, and histamine. J Allergy Clin Immunol 1990;85:856–8.

[6] Slater EE, Merrill DD, Guess HA, et al. Clinical profile of angioedema associated with angiotensin converting-enzyme inhibition. JAMA 1988;260:967–70.

[7] Venable RJ. Angioedema after long-term enalapril use. J Fam Prac 1992;34:201–4.

[8] Irons BK, Kumar A. Valsartan induced angioedema. Ann Pharmacother 2003;37:1024–7.

[9] Cicardi M, Zingale LC, Bergamaschini L, et al. Angioedema associated with angiotensin-converting enzyme inhibitor use: outcome after switching to a different treatment. Arch Intern Med 2004;26:910–3.

[10] Cochran ST. Anaphylactoid reactions to radiocontrast media. Curr Allergy Asthma Rep 2005;5:28–31.

[11] Setkowicz M, Zembowicz A, Mastalerz L, et al. Non-steroidal anti-inflammatory drugs (NSAID) sensitivity in chronic idiophatic urticaria CIU: selective involvement of cyclooxygenase 1 (COX-1) and overproduction of cysteinyl-leukotrienes. J Allergy Clin Immunol 2003;111:S272.

[12] Bork K, Fischer B, Dewald G. Recurrent episodes of skin angioedema and severe attacks of abdominal pain induced by oral contraceptives or hormone replacement therapy. Am J Med 2003;114:294–8.

[13] Leiferman KM, Gleich GJ. Hypereosinophilic syndrome: case presentation and update. J Allergy Clin Immunol 2004;113:50–8.

[14] Kazmierowski JA, Chusid MJ, Parillo JE, et al. Dermtologic manifestations of the hypereosinophilic syndrome. Arch Dermatol 1978;114:531–5.

[15] Gleich GJ, Schroeter AL, Marcoux JP, et al. Episodic angioedema associated with eosinophilia. N Engl J Med 1984;310:1621–6.

[16] Chikama R, Hosokawa M, Miyazawa T, et al. Nonepisodic angioedema associated with eosinophilia: report of 4 cases and review of 33 young female patients reported in Japan. Dermatology 1998;197:321–5.

[17] Mascaro JM. Other vesiculobullous diseases. In: Bolognia JL, Jorizzo JL, Rapini RP, editors. Dermatology. London: Mosby; 2003. p. 501–8.

[18] Rice TW, Rodriguez RM, Light RW. The superior vena cava syndrome: clinical characteristics and evolving etiology. Medicine (Baltimore) 2006;85:37–42.

[19] Kestler A, Keyes I. Images in clinical medicine. Quincke's edema. N Engl J Med 2003;349: 867.

[20] Corazza M, Pizzigoni S, Sprocati M, et al. Acute idiopathic scrotal edema in children. Dermatology 2003;206:343–4.

[21] Van Dellen RG, Maddox DE, Dutta EJ. Masqueraders of angioedema and urticaria. Ann Allergy Asthma Immunol 2002;88:10–5.

[22] Miyagawa S, Takahashi Y, Nagai A, et al. Angio-oedema in a neonate with IgG antibodies to parvovirus B19 following intrauterine parvovirus B19 following intrauterine parvovirus B19 infection. Br J Dermatol 2000;143:428–30.

[23] Wisnieski J, Jones S. Comparison of autoantibodies to the collagen-like region of C1q in hypocomplementemic urticarial vasculitis syndrome and systemic lupus erythematosus. J Immunol 1992;148:1396–403.

[24] Saigal K, Valencia IC, Cohen J, et al. Hypocomplementemic urticarial vasculitis with angioedema, a rare presentation of systemic lupus erythematosus: rapid resonse to rituximab. J Am Acad Dermatol 2003;49:S283–5.

[25] Wang HP, Huang CC, Chen CH, et al. Weber-Christian disease presenting with intractable fever and periorbital swelling mimicking angioedema. Clin Rheumatol 2006 [Epub ahead of print].

[26] Lamprecht P, Moosig F, Adam-Klages S, et al. Small vessel vasculitis and relapsing panniculitis in tumour necrosis factor receptor associated periodic syndrome (TRAPS). Ann Rheum Dis 2004;63:1518–20.

[27] Heymann WR. Cutaneous manifestations of thyroid disease. J Am Acad Dermatol 1992;39: 846–9.

[28] Rebora A, Rongioletti F. Mucinoses. In: Bolognia JL, Jorizzo JL, Rapini RP, editors. Dermatology. London: Mosby; 2003. p. 647–58.

[29] Rongioletti F, Rebora A. Updated classification of papular mucinosis, lichen myxedematosus, and scleromyxedema. J Am Acad Dermatol 2001;44:273–81.

[30] Kyle RA, Gertz MA. Primary systemic amyloidosis: clinical and laboratory features in 474 cases. Smin Hematol 1995;32:45–59.

[31] Brehmer-Andersson E, Kaaman T, Skog E, et al. The histopathogenesis of the flame figure in Wells' syndrome based on five cases. Acta Derm Venereol 1986;66:213–9.

[32] Lakhanpal S, Ginsburg WW, Michet CJ, et al. Eosinophilic fasciitis: clinical spectrum and therapeutic response in 52 cases. Semin Arthritis Rheumatol 1998;17:221–31.

[33] Gordon ML, Lebowohl MG, Phelps RG, et al. Eosinophilic fasciitis associated with tryptophan ingestion: a manifestation of eosinophilic myalgia syndrome. Arch Dermatol 1991;127: 217–20.

[34] Lityakova LI, Bellanti JA. Orofacial edema: a diagnostic and therapeutic challenge for the clinician. Ann Allergy Asthma Immunol 2000;84:188–92.

[35] Cocuroccia B, Gubinelli E, Annessi G, et al. Persistent unilateral orbital and eyelid oedema as a manifestation of Melkersson-Rosenthal syndrome. J Eur Acad Dermatol Venereol 2005; 19:107–11.

[36] Allen CM, Camisa C, Hamzeh S, et al. Cheilitis granulomatosa: report of six cases and review of the literature. J Am Acad Dermatol 1990;23:444–50.

[37] Bogenrieder T, Rogler G, Vogt T, et al. Orofacial granulomatosis as the initial presentation of Crohn's disease in an adolescent. Dermatology 2003;206:273–8.

[38] Schwartzbauer HR, Tami TA. Ear, nose, and throat manifestations of sarcoidosis. Otolaryngol Clin North Amer 2003;36:673–84.

[39] Cohen DM, Green JM, Diekmann SL. Concurrent anomalies: cheilitis glandularis and double lip: a report of a case. Oral Surg Oral Med Oral Pathol 1988;66:397–9.

[40] Ioannidou DI, Krasagakis K, Stefanidou MP, et al. Scleredema adultorum of Buschke presenting as periorbital edema: a diagnostic challenge. J Am Acad Dermatol 2005;52:41–4.

[41] Custer PL, Tenzel RR, Kowalzyck AP. Blepharochalasis syndrome. Am J Ophthalmol 1985; 99:424–8.

[42] Cicardi M, Zingale LC, Pappalardo E, et al. Autoantibodies and lymphoproliferative diseases in acquired C1-inhibitor deficiencies. Medicine 2003;82:274–81.

[43] Vella FS, Panella E, Masciale N, et al. Clarkson syndrome: a rare clinical condition characterized by generalized edema associated to monoclonal gammopathy. Recenti Prog Med 2005;96:488–91.

[44] Auricchio L, Vitiello L, Adriani M, et al. Cutaneous manifestations as presenting sign of autoimmune lymphoproliferative syndrome in childhood. Dermatology 2005;210:336–40.

[45] Drappa J, Vaishnaw AK, Sullivan K, et al. FAS gene mutations in the Canale-Smith, an inherited lymphoproliferative disorder associated with autoimmunity. N Engl J Med 1996; 335:1643–9.

[46] Cunningham BB, Caro WA, Eramo LR. Neonatal acute hemorrhagic edema of childhood: case report and review of the English-language literature. Pediatr Dermatol 1996;13:39–44.

[47] Kaplan AP, Greaves MW. Angioedema. J Am Acad Dermatol 2005;53:373–88.

ELSEVIER
SAUNDERS

Immunol Allergy Clin N Am
26 (2006) 615–632

IMMUNOLOGY
AND ALLERGY
CLINICS
OF NORTH AMERICA

Structure and Function of C1-Inhibitor

Ineke G.A. Wagenaar-Bos, PhD[a],*,
C. Erik Hack, MD, PhD[b,c]

[a]*Department of Immunopathology, Sanquin Research at CLB and Landsteiner Laboratory,*
Academical Medical Center, University of Amsterdam, Plesmanlaan 125,
1066 CX Amsterdam, the Netherlands
[b]*Crucell Nederland NV, P.O. Box 2048, 2301 CA, Leiden, the Netherlands*
[c]*Department of Clinical Chemistry, VU Medical Center, Amsterdam, the Netherlands*

Hereditary angioedema (HAE) is an autosomal dominant inheritable disorder that is caused by a heterozygous deficiency in the plasma protein, C1-inhibitor (C1-INH). The role of C1-INH deficiency in HAE was first identified in the early 1960s [1,2]. C1-INH is a plasma protein that inhibits proteases of both the coagulation system and the complement system, thereby inhibiting different inflammatory and coagulant pathways. C1-INH consists of two domains, a C-terminal and an N-terminal domain. The C-terminal domain clearly shows the features of a serine protease inhibitor (serpin), a class of proteins with diverse functions and a highly conserved structure throughout evolution. The N-terminal domain has a unique sequence not sharing homology with any known protein. To understand the structure and the mechanism of action of C1-INH, the general structure and function of serpins is described first, followed by a more specific description of C1-INH.

Serpin structure and function

Serine proteinase inhibitors (serpins) are characterized by a typical structure and mechanism of action, which may be summarized as a suicide inhibitor that traps the protease as a kind of set mousetrap. The main function of serpins is to inhibit serine proteases, although some serpins can regulate activity of other proteases as well [3]. The preferred protease to be inhibited by

---

* Corresponding author. Department of Immunopathology, Sanquin Research at CLB, Plesmanlaan 125, 1066 CX Amsterdam, the Netherlands.
E-mail address: i.bos@sanquin.nl (I.G.A. Wagenaar-Bos).

0889-8561/06/$ - see front matter © 2006 Elsevier Inc. All rights reserved.
doi:10.1016/j.iac.2006.08.004   *immunology.theclinics.com*

a serpin is called the target protease. Though most serpins have one target protease, C1-INH has several (see further discussion). Serpins inhibit serine proteases by formation of stable equimolar complexes. The crystal structure of several serpins has been solved, generating basic knowledge of serpin structure [4–7]. All serpins are made up of three β-sheets, surrounded by eight or nine α-helices and a protruding reactive site loop (Fig. 1). The reactive site is located on the outside of the molecule, on the flexible reactive site loop, which is free to interact with target proteases. Key residues are the so-called "P1 and P1'" residues, which are recognized by the target protease as a substrate.

Serpin structure is highly conserved throughout evolution: all serpins share the complex template structure that has the unusual property of undergoing gross conformational changes [8]. Approximately 500 serpins of all different organisms have been identified by sequence similarity. Serpins are known as suicide substrates for the protease. The active form of the

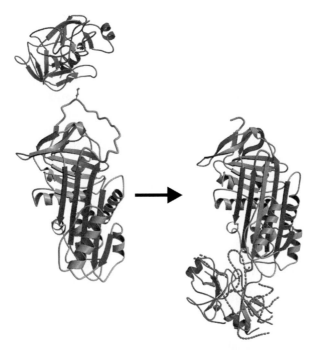

Fig. 1. Formation of the complex of serpin and protease. Ribbon depictions of native α1-antitrypsin with trypsin aligned above in the docking orientation (*left*) and of the complex showing the 7.1-nm shift of the P1 methionine of α1-antitrypsin, with full insertion of the cleaved reactive center loop into the central β-sheet. Regions of disordered structure in the complexed trypsin are shown as interrupted coils projected from the native structure of trypsin. Red, α1-antitrypsin in the central β-sheet; yellow, reactive site loop; green ball and stick, P1 Met; cyan, trypsin (with helices in magenta for orientation); red ball and stick, active serine 195. (*From* Huntington JA, Read RJ, Carrell RW. Structure of a serpin-protease complex shows inhibition by deformation. Nature 2000;407(6806):924; with permission.)

serpin is a set mousetrap, with the ability to trap the protease as soon as the protease binds and cleaves the P1–P1' peptidyl bond in the reactive center. Subsequently, the reactive site loop is inserted into the central β-sheet, thereby moving 7.1 nm to the opposite side of the serpin, while still being covalently bound by its P1-residue to the active site serine of the protease [9]. The driving force for this dramatic conformational change is an affinity-based insertion of the reactive site loop (P15–P1) into the hydrophobic core of the central β-sheet. Tight binding of the serpin to the protease leads to distortion of the catalytic triad of the protease, which prevents completion of the proteolytic reaction [10]. As a consequence, the active site of the protease remains bound to the P1-residue of the inserted reactive site loop. In this way, covalently linked complexes of the serpin and its target protease are formed in which the active site of the protease is blocked.

For the interaction between α1-antitrypsin and trypsin, it has been suggested that distortion of the complete protease in the complex is an integral part of the inhibition process, because 37% of the protease structure was crystallographically disordered [9]. This changed conformation of the protease renders it more susceptible to proteolytic attack by other proteases. However, no such complete distortion was observed in a complex between α1-antitrypsin and porcine pancreatic elastase, suggesting that distortion of the active site of the protease alone is sufficient for inhibition and that enhanced proteolysis of the protease is not necessarily exploited in vivo [11].

Conformational changes involving insertion of the reactive site loop in the central β-sheet may also occur in conditions different from protease inhibition. Because serpins operate by a typical branched pathway [12], cleavage of the serpin as well as stable complex formation can occur, depending on the characteristics of the serpin (Fig. 2) [13].

Flexibility of the so-called "hinge region," at the start of the reactive site loop (Fig. 3), is essential to efficient trapping. When trapping is insufficient, the serpin is cleaved by the protease, while the loop is inserted into the central β-sheet, but the protease is released from the loop before its catalytic site becomes distorted. This released protease retains its proteolytic activity. Insufficient trapping can occur when the serpin is attacked by a nontarget protease or in the case of certain pathologic mutations in the serpin, as

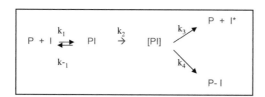

Fig. 2. The branched pathway of serpins. P, protease; I, serpin; I*, cleaved inhibitor. PI and [PI] are intermediate stages of the serpin-protease complex. For more information, see Brown EW, Ravindran S, Patston PA. The reaction between plasmin and C1-inhibitor results in plasmin inhibition by the serpin mechanism. Blood Coagul Fibrinolysis 2002;13(8):711–4.

Reactive site ⟹

Hinge region

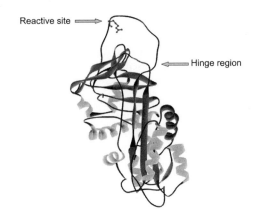

Fig. 3. Three-dimensional model of the structure of the serpin domain of C1-INH. (*From* Bos IG, Hack CE, Abrahams SP. Structural and functional aspects of C1-inhibitor. Immunobiology 2002;205(4–5):518–33; with permission.)

described in a later section. These two different outcomes of an interaction between a protease and a serpin are described as the branched pathway of serpins (see Fig. 2). In addition, two other interactions between reactive site loop and the central β-sheet may occur that do not require proteolytic cleavage of the former. First spontaneous insertion of the reactive site loop (ie, without cleavage by a protease) into the central β-sheet may occur in some serpins, yielding the so-called "latent conformation." Another possible interaction is intermolecular polymerization by means of so-called "loop–sheet linkage": the reactive site loop of one molecule inserts into the β-sheet of another molecule. Latency and multimerization are closely linked, because they both result from a destabilized central β-sheet. Conversion to the cleaved, latent, or loop-sheet multimer conformation results in increased thermal stability of the serpin and loss of inhibitory activity [14]. It is suggested that latent and cleaved conformations of various serpins may serve other physiologic functions [15].

In human plasma, many different serpins involved in inhibition of inflammation and coagulation are known. As of 2002, 34 human serpins had been identified [16] that together form the principal inhibitors controlling both intracellular and extracellular proteolytic pathways. For example, antithrombin controls coagulation, the inhibitors of plasmin and its activators control fibrinolysis, and α1-antitrypsin inhibits neutrophil elastase as well as trypsin.

Structure of the serpin domain of C1-inhibitor

Mature C1-INH is a protein of 478 amino acids and is heavily glycosylated; indeed, C1-INH appears so far to be the largest known serpin [17]. On sodium dodecyl sulfate polyacrylamide gel electrophoresis

(SDS-PAGE) it migrates with an apparent molecular weight (MW) of 104 kDa, although the calculated MW is 76 kDa with glycans and 53 kDa without glycans. C1-INH consists of a serpin domain of 365 amino acids and an N-terminal nonserpin domain of 113 amino acids. The amino acid sequence of the serpin domain shows clear homology to that of other serpins. Based on this homology, a three-dimensional model of its structure has been made [18], which is shown in Fig. 3.

Some remarkable features of the serpin domain of C1-INH are (1) its short reactive site loop compared with other serpins [19]; (2) a suggested secondary binding site for one of its target proteases, C1s [20]; and (3) its glycosylation on three different residues (residue numbers 216, 231, and 330), next to extensive glycosylation on 10 residues of the N-terminal domain, resulting in a total of 13 glycosylation sites that compose approximately 30% of the weight of C1-INH.

The short reactive site loop, though exceptional, is not unique to C1-INH, given that CrmA has a similar short reactive site loop. The reactive site loop length is probably important for efficient distortion of the catalytic triad of the protease on trapping, but the functional implication of the short version in C1-INH is still unknown.

The structure of the unique N-terminal domain of C1-INH has not yet been elucidated. Although attempts to crystallize C1-INH have been made, these have not succeeded, because of failure to obtain sufficiently large diffractable crystals (possibly resulting from the extensive glycosylation of C1-INH). One other interesting feature of C1-INH structure is the disulfide linkage between the N-terminal and the serpin domain by means of cysteine residues linking 101 to 406 and 108 to 183.

Based on observations with a C1-INH mutant isolated from a patient who had HAE, the authors have demonstrated that loss of this disulfide bridge resulted in a multimerized conformation. This conformation may have been due to loop–sheet linkage, because it was definitely not due to disulfide linkage of molecules, and the resulting mutant showed increased heat stability and reactivity with monoclonal antibody's (mAb) specific for the loop-inserted conformation [21]. This finding demonstrates a stabilizing function of the N-terminal domain for the central β-sheet of the serpin domain of C1-INH, resembling the stabilizing effect of heparin on antithrombin III, both essential to maintenance of the metastable conformation.

Function of C1-inhibitor

Target proteases

C1-INH is the major inhibitor of the classical pathway of the complement system and is also known as an inhibitor of coagulation. C1-INH has several target proteinases, including factor XIIa [22,23], kallikrein

[24,25], and factor XIa [26] of the contact system, activated C1s and C1r of the classical pathway [27–29], and the proteinases of the mannose binding lectin (MBL) pathway (MASP) of complement [30] (see article elsewhere in this issue for more details). C1-INH may be considered an inhibitor of different inflammatory pathways, although the physiologic relevance of the interaction with the MASPs in vivo is still unclear, given that no kinetic data are available. The P1-P1′ residues of C1-INH are arginine and threonine, respectively. An arginine at P1 predicts specificity for trypsin-like proteases, which indeed matches the specificity of the target proteases. Mutants with cysteine or histidine at the P1 position are dysfunctional and have been described in patients who have type II HAE [31]. The protease specificity is also determined by the residues around P1. For example, mutations at the P2 position, Ala443, also influence target protease recognition. Mutation of Ala443 to Val diminishes the inhibitory activity of C1-INH toward C1s and C1r, although this mutant protein can inhibit trypsin and has normal interaction with kallikrein and XIIa [32,33]. The locations of other interaction sites on the C1-INH molecule are not well known, except for one site (Gln452-Phe455) involved in the interaction with C1s [20]. The importance of this secondary binding site for C1s has, however, been challenged by a study showing that mutation of the residues 452 and 453 to alanine had no effect on the association rates of C1-INH with C1s and did not impair complex formation between C1-INH and C1s, C1r, kallikrein, or XIIa [34].

C1-INH is also described as inhibiting porcine chymotrypsin [35], plasmin [13], and thrombin [36]. The physiologic relevance of these interactions is, however, unclear, because other, more potent inhibitors are also present in plasma, and plasmin activation, for example, does not result in a decrease in active C1-INH levels. Besides inhibiting the classical pathway of complement, C1-INH has recently been demonstrated to inhibit the alternative pathway as well [37].

Hinge region

Like all serpins, C1-INH undergoes conformational changes on interaction with the target protease, resulting from insertion of part of the reactive site loop. In particular, the amino acid residues P14 to P10 in the hinge region (see Fig. 3) are important for rapid formation of a conformation-altered C1-INH, which is tightly bound to the target proteinase. The importance of the residues at P14, P12, and P10 for the conformational changes and for the inhibitory function is underscored by their high degree of conservation in serpins. Furthermore, mutations of these residues have been described in some patients who have HAE, leading to a dysfunctional C1-INH protein [38] (and reviewed by Davis [39]). Disturbed flexibility of this hinge region decelerates insertion of the reactive site loop on protease binding, allowing the protease to cleave the serpin before being trapped.

Inhibitory activity

The inhibitory activity of C1-INH is low compared with that of other serpins, as demonstrated by a relatively slow association constant of C1-INH with its target proteases. The association rate constants are 6×10^4 $M^{-1}s^{-1}$, 0.8×10^4 $M^{-1}s^{-1}$, and 0.4×10^3 $M^{-1}s^{-1}$ for C1-INH with C1s, kallikrein, and factor XIIa, respectively, compared with 10^7 $M^{-1}s^{-1}$ for α1-antitrypsin with neutrophil elastase [40] (and summarized in [16]). The most likely explanation for this is a diminished exposure of the reactive site, possibly resulting from the short reactive site loop. C1-INH traps its target proteases efficiently, because the stoichiometry of this interaction is 1.05 at 38°C [12]. All the association constants described earlier have been determined with purified proteins. Interestingly, C1 bound to larger immune complexes is much less efficiently inactivated than is C1 bound to smaller immune complexes, and C1 bound to the surface of sensitized sheep erythrocytes requires as much as 100-fold more C1-INH for inactivation than does the same amount of fluid-phase active C1 [41,42].

Potentiation by glycosaminoglycans

The function of C1-INH may be markedly enhanced by glycosaminoglycans (GAG), such as heparin and the semisynthetic dextran sulfate [43,44]. The mechanism of potentiation of antithrombin III by heparin has been well defined. It comprises expulsion of the reactive site loop, which is pushed out of the central β-sheet, resulting in improved exposure of the reactive site. It may be concluded from our three-dimensional model that this mechanism cannot explain potentiation of C1-INH, because the reactive site loop of C1-INH is five amino acids shorter than that of antithrombin III. The D-helix is the major binding site for heparin to antithrombin, but the D-helix in C1-INH is short compared with that of antithrombin III, as well. The binding site for GAG on C1-INH is not known, nor is the mechanism of potentiation. Strikingly, C1-INH can only be potentiated toward the target proteases C1s and factor XIa and not toward factor XIIa or kallikrein, although a 1.4-fold enhancement of the inhibition of kallikrein has been described [45]. However, the authors believe that 1.4-fold enhancement is not a convincing potentiation compared with the 70- to 100-fold enhancement toward factor XIa and C1s [43,44]. This specific potentiation suggests involvement of sites specific for C1s and XIa in potentiation, but such involvement has not been proved so far. Another interesting, but completely different, potentiating factor has been described. The *Escherichia coli* O157:H7–derived metalloprotease StcE cleaves C1-INH in the heavily glycosylated N-terminal domain and appears to form a bridge between the complement activating agent and C1-INH to increase efficient localization of C1-INH and subsequent inhibition [46].

Administration of exogenous glycosaminoglycans to potentiate C1-INH in vivo yielded variable results. Administration of heparin or N-acetyl heparin in cardiac ischemia reperfusion in canine or rabbit hearts resulted in a decrease in myocardial dysfunction secondary to ischemia reperfusion [47,48], which may be related to C1-INH potentiation or complement inhibition in vivo. By contrast, a clinical trial of inhaled and subcutaneous heparin in patients who had HAE failed to prevent exacerbations of angioedema [49]. This may be a simple result of remaining C1-INH levels in these patients being too low for significant potentiation. However, it should be realized that C1-INH can only be potentiated to inhibit factor XIa and C1s and not toward the contact system proteases factor XIIa and kallikrein. When these proteases are the prevailing effectors in an HAE attack, heparin will not modify its course.

The physiologic relevance of potentiation by glycosaminoglycans is not clear. The authors assume that C1-INH is potentiated on binding to heparan sulfate on the endothelium. This process would facilitate localization of the enhanced inhibition onto the endothelium. Recently, heparan sulfate has been shown to play a role in the entry of leukocytes at sites of inflammation [50]; variation in heparan sulfate structure under normal and inflammatory conditions has been postulated as a regulatory mechanism for chemokine binding. Similarly, variations in potentiation of C1-INH at inflammatory sites in vivo may be envisaged.

The N-terminal domain of C1-inhibitor

C1-INH has a unique N-terminal domain consisting of 116 amino acids. The two cysteine residues located near the C-terminus of this domain, Cys101 and Cys108, form disulfide bridges with two cysteines in the serpin domain, Cys406 and Cys183, respectively. These two disulfide bridges stabilize the metastable conformation of the serpin domain [21]. The association and dissociation constants, as well as complex formation on SDS-PAGE with several target proteases, were not affected by removal of the first 98 amino acids of the N-terminal domain [21,51], indicating that it has a minor role in inhibition of the target proteases in vitro. A recent publication, however, describes an inhibiting effect of the N-terminal domain on the inhibition of kallikrein. In the presence of endothelial cells, 1 µM of C1-INH was needed to inhibit 3 nM of kallikrein. The requirement of a large molar excess of C1-INH was not observed when part of the C1-INH N-terminal domain was cleaved by the StcE metalloproteinase, a finding that suggests a novel regulatory function of this domain with regard to the inhibition kinetics in the presence of cells [52]. However, this article also demonstrated an increased interaction rate with kallikrein after cleavage with StcE, whereas the authors have not observed any effect of deleting the N-terminal domain of C1-INH on the interaction with kallikrein under pseudo–first-order conditions [21]. Hence the precise role of the N-terminal domain on the inhibition kinetics is still not definitively established.

Recent studies by A. Davis and coworkers [53] have shed some light on a possible novel function of the N-terminal domain of C1-INH. In a series of experiments, these investigators have demonstrated that C1-INH is able to bind lipopolysaccharide (LPS) of some bacteria, which effect was dependent on the presence of the N-terminal domain. This effect is proposed as a partial explanation of the beneficial effects of C1-INH in sepsis. Further studies indicated that binding to LPS is dependent on Asn3, which contains an N-linked glycan, and on four positively charged amino acids within the amino-terminal domain (ie, Arg18, Lys22, Lys30, and Lys55), each of which had an additive effect on the binding [54].

Glycosylation

C1-INH contains 13 glycosylation sites. Removal of the N-terminal domain, which contains 10 of the 13 glycosylation sites, has no effect either on the formation of SDS-stable complexes with target proteases [51] or on the association rate constant with the target proteases C1s, XIIa, and kallikrein [21]. Deglycosylation of plasma C1-INH with N-glycanase, O-glycanase, or both also has no major effect on C1-INH function. Moreover, removal of sialic acid groups does not affect inhibition of C4 activation by C1s [55]. Desialylated C1-INH is still able to form complexes with C1s [56]. The kinetics of the interaction of a nonglycosylated variant have not been determined so far, but the data suggest that the glycosylation does not affect serpin activity toward the best-known target proteases. A different glycosylation pattern, occurring when C1-INH is produced in the yeast *Pichia pastoris* or in the milk of transgenic rabbits, does not affect inhibition of several target proteases [40,57]. It appears probable, however, that the glycosylation of Asn231 affects the stability of the central β-sheet and consequently that glycosylation may play a subtle role in protease trapping and the binding kinetics.

Glycosylation does have a significant effect on the plasma half-life of C1-INH. Removal of the ultimate sialic acid groups from C1-INH enhances the clearance rate by the liver in a rabbit model [55], probably by binding of desialylated C1-INH to hepatic asialoglycoprotein receptors. Subsequent removal of the penultimate galactose residues results in clearance rates near normal. A different glycosylation pattern, as on human recombinant C1-INH produced in the yeast *P pastoris* [40] or in milk from transgenic rabbits [57], also leads to enhanced clearance rates.

By contrast, different glycosylation may play a role in a compensatory mechanism in patients who have HAE, as has been described by Zhang and colleagues [58]. Comparison of C1-INH glycans from normal individuals with those of patients who had HAE demonstrated identical O-glycan structures but different N-glycans in patients who had HAE, in that these glycans were small, were highly charged, and lacked sialidase-releasable N-acetylneuraminic acid. The different charges may result from the presence of mannose-6-phosphate residues. These residues might facilitate secretion of C1-INH through an alternative lysosomal pathway, possibly serving as a compensatory mechanism to enhance plasma levels of C1-INH in these deficient patients. The half-life of this C1-INH variant is still to be determined, but the paper suggests an interesting role for glycosylation in synthesis.

Several studies have shown that glycosylated acute-phase proteins during acute-phase reactions may bear sialyl-Lewis[x] moieties, which allow these proteins to interact with E- and P-selectins on the endothelium and to attenuate adherence of leukocytes to it [59,60]. The presence of these moieties has also been demonstrated on C1-INH, which explains the inhibitory effect of this serpin on leukocyte-endothelium adhesion [61]. This interesting feature endows C1-INH with the property of protecting endothelium during inflammatory conditions, which may explain the anti-inflammatory effect of this protein.

Effect of mutations on C1-inhibitor function

More than 100 different mutations have been identified in patients who have HAE ("every family has its own mutation"), all sharing the property of resulting in low levels of functional C1-INH protein in the circulation. These mutations involve large deletions, nonsense mutations, or missense mutations (resulting in the expression of a dysfunctional protein). This article only describes the mutations leading to dysfunctional protein. Regulatory mutations, nonsense mutations, or frame shifts result in low levels of C1-INH by obvious mechanisms. Mutations leading to dysfunctional protein, however, can illustrate the amino acid residues important for C1-INH function and may reveal unexpectedly important sites.

C1-INH deficiency is inherited as an autosomal dominant disorder, and no homozygous patients have been described so far. Unfortunately, no thorough analysis of occurring polymorphisms has been performed yet, and only two polymorphisms are known: Gln165Glu (P05155 in Protein Database) and Val 458Met [17].

In the human gene mutation database [62] and the HAE database [63], mutations of 55 amino acids leading to HAE have been described. Of these residues, 21 are conserved and 10 are semiconserved residues. All these mutations reside in the serpin domain. Interestingly, no mutations in the unique N-terminal domain have been described thus far, suggesting that mutations in this region do not result in HAE. This finding is in line with experiments in which deletion of the first 98 amino acids has no effect on inhibitory activity [21,51]. Only the two cysteines linking the serpin domain with the unique N-terminal domain have a major role in stabilization of the central β-sheet [21].

A variety of different missense mutations and small deletions or insertions lead to different dysfunctional conformations of C1-INH. As for all serpins, three types of mutations may be described at the structural level, leading to (1) a molecule with altered exposure of the reactive site, (2) cleavage of C1-INH at the reactive site, or (3) latency or multimerization. Note that this classification of dysfunctional C1-INH proteins does not correspond to the type I:type II dichotomy of HAE.

In type I HAE, low levels of both antigen and functional C1-INH are detected in plasma, whereas in type II HAE, low levels of functional C1-INH are accompanied by normal levels of C1-INH antigen. Type I HAE can be caused by mutations leading to deficient C1-INH synthesis, as well as by mutations leading to impaired secretion of a dysfunctional protein (for example, caused by intracellular multimerization or aggregation). In type II HAE, cleaved, inert, or latent C1-INH mutant molecules may occur. Typically, less than 50% of the level of functional C1-INH is found in patients who are heterozygous for the mutation. Excessive consumption of normal C1-INH has been mentioned as a possible explanation.

Many different mutations have been described in the last decade, but, of the 55 amino acids that are mutated in patients who have HAE, only 13 mutants have been investigated thoroughly enough to provide explanations for the dysfunction. Regarding the other residues involved in HAE mutants, only speculations about their structural impact may be made [18]. Here the authors limit the discussion to mutations whose functional consequences can be understood in light of the known structure and mechanism of serpins in general and C1-INH in particular. These are discussed based on the three categories described earlier.

Category I mutations lead to an inert C1-INH molecule or an inhibitor with a different protease specificity. These mutations usually occur as a consequence of altered composition or exposure of the reactive site. Category I contains several interesting mutants. Mutations in the reactive site loop typically lead to altered protease recognition. Mutation of P1 Arg444 to Cys demonstrates 75% and 50% inhibition of C1s and kallikrein, respectively, but enhanced inhibition of factor XII [31]. Mutation of Arg444 to His results in a better inhibitor of chymotrypsin than normal C1-INH [64]. Arg444Leu (which shows a phenotype intermediate between type I and type II HAE) demonstrates no cleaved C1-INH on SDS-PAGE but increased elastase susceptibility, pointing to altered protease specificity [65]. Mutation of the P2, Ala 443 to Val, diminishes the inhibition of C1s and C1r, while enhancing inhibition of trypsin and demonstrating a normal interaction with XIIa and kallikrein [33]. Mutation of Ala 443 to Asp, which has a bulky and charged side chain, results in defective inhibition of C1r and XIIa, as well as impaired inhibition of C1s and kallikrein [32]. This mutant further supports the hypothesis that the interaction of C1-INH with its target proteases is in part dependent on different amino acid residues. This hypothesis is also supported by the observation that potentiation by heparin is observed only toward XIa and C1s and not toward factor XIIa and kallikrein. Other interesting mutants in the reactive site loop are mutants of the P3 and P5 residues that are resistant to catalytic inactivation by human neutrophil elastase, while inhibitory capacity is not affected [64]. However, these mutants do not occur in vivo but have been synthesized in a recombinant system.

Protease specificity is mainly related to the conformation of the reactive site loop. Hence, the mutations that lead to an impaired interaction with certain proteases probably influence the accessibility of the reactive site. Most striking is the ability of the Ala 443–Val mutation to inhibit trypsin. Wild-type C1-INH scarcely inhibits trypsin; rather, it is primarily inactivated by this protease. Apparently, trypsin efficiently cleaves the peptidyl bond between Arg at P1 and Thr at P1′, and it completes hydrolysis of this peptidyl bond before complete insertion of the reactive site loop in the central sheet. It may be speculated that in the case of the Ala 443–Val mutant, hydrolysis of the peptidyl bond is less efficient, leaving sufficient time for the trapping mechanism of the inhibitor. In other words, the insertion of the reactive site loop of the mutant is completed before the bond between the active site serine of trypsin and Arg at P1 is hydrolyzed. Consequently, the catalytic triad of trypsin becomes disturbed while the active site serine is still bound to Arg 444, and the complex between trypsin and C1-INH is stabilized.

Category II mutations lead to enhanced cleavage of C1-INH, resulting from inefficient trapping after protease binding. Mutations in the hinge region are of special interest for category II mutants. The ability to keep the protease trapped is reflected by the dissociation constant (k_{off}). In theory, a molecule with a very high k_{on} and a very high k_{off} is not an inhibitor but rather a suitable substrate. Mutations in the hinge region of C1-INH (P14, P12, and P10) convert C1-INH into a substrate for its target proteases, probably because the docking of the reactive site loop of these mutants into the central sheet is too slow, which impairs the trapping of the protease. While several P1 mutations have been described as causing the aforementioned category I mutants, many different mutations of the reactive site have been described (particularly those of P1 Arg 444). It appears likely that the P1 mutations include mutations that lead to enhanced cleavage of the molecule. All of the described mutations at P1 lead to type II HAE, with normal antigenic levels of C1-INH and low functional levels [31,65–67]. Obviously, both a C1-INH molecule inert toward target proteases (category I) and a cleaved molecule (category II) will lead to this diagnosis. For the mutants Arg444His and Arg444Cys, it is clear that they belong to category I. Of Arg444Pro not much is known, and for Arg444Ser and Arg 444Leu no cleaved C1-INH was observed in patient plasma on SDS-PAGE [66,67].

Category III mutations lead to a latent conformation or loop-sheet multimers, resulting from spontaneous insertion of the reactive site loop into the central β-sheet of the same or an adjacent molecule. Deletion of Lys251 leads to multimerization of C1-INH and converts the molecule into a substrate [68]. Deletion of this residue results in a new glycosylation site. However, the dysfunction of this mutant could not be attributed to the presence of an additional carbohydrate group, because production of this mutant in the presence of tunicamycin did not restore function. Deletion of Lys251 is likely to disrupt the structure of the central β-sheet, because this amino acid is located in a loop overlying the central β-sheet. This mutant formed no complexes with C1s, C1r, or kallikrein and formed complexes inefficiently with factor XIIa. Each of the proteases induced partial cleavage on the mutant inhibitor, indicating insufficiency of the trapping mechanism (category II).

Another mutation at P10 from Ala to Thr results in blocked protease recognition and polymerization of the molecule (category III) [69]. Mutations in the C-terminal region of the reactive site loop at the conserved residues Val 451, Phe 455, and Pro 476 also lead to multimerization. This effect is probably due to deterioration of anchoring of the reactive site loop, resulting in overinsertion of the loop into the central β-sheet, which subsequently leads to multimerization (category III) [70,71]. All these residues are located in β-sheet C, between the central β-sheet (A) and the reactive site loop. Several other mutations in the C-terminal region of C1-INH (Phe 457 Leu and Met 470 Lys) have been reported in patients who have HAE. Whether these mutations result in reduced production of C1-INH or in a dysfunction of the molecule is, however, not known [72].

The structure-to-function relationships gleaned from the analysis of well-characterized C1-INH mutations follow predictable patterns, as described in the following discussion. Mutations in the reactive site lead to type II HAE, resulting from an inert molecule that cannot react with target proteases, a cleaved molecule, or a molecule with altered interactions. All these variations are due to altered exposure of the reactive site. Mutations in the hinge region lead to either type I or type II HAE. Type II HAE in this case is the result of inefficient trapping, due to diminished flexibility of the hinge region or blocked interaction with the target protease. Type I HAE can be the result of polymerization of the molecule due to diminished anchoring of the reactive site loop, which leads to diminished secretion resulting from intracellular accumulation or degradation of C1-INH. Mutations in very diverse parts of the C1-INH molecule can lead to altered stability of the central β-sheet and thus to multimerization of the molecule, generally resulting in type I HAE. Many of the mutants described in this category reside in the sheet C, which is located behind the central β-sheet, and one mutant misses the disulphide bridges linking the N-terminal with the serpin domain of C1-INH.

Autoantibodies to C1-inhibitor

After recognition that HAE can be caused by a genetic deficiency of C1-INH, it was discovered that some patients suffered from an acquired form of angioedema (AAE), which is generally associated with the presence of an autoimmune or a lymphoproliferative disorder. Levels of functional C1-INH in this disease typically are very low, although antigenic levels may be higher, suggesting the presence of a nonfunctional C1-INH molecule in the circulation. Indeed, some studies have shown that patients who have AAE have a circulating C1-INH with a lower MW than functional C1-INH [73,74]. In addition, autoantibodies against C1-INH are frequently detected in plasma samples from patients who have AAE, suggesting that the decrease in levels of functional C1-INH results from the presence of autoantibodies [75]. Theoretically, such antibodies may reduce C1-INH levels by multiple mechanisms, such as enhanced clearance due to uptake by Fc-receptors carrying cells or covering functional sites on the molecule. However, most evidence in the literature points to another mechanism: several investigators have shown that addition of autoantibodies to functional C1-INH results in impaired complex formation with and enhanced cleavage by target proteases, such as C1s [74,76,77]. The epitopes for these antibodies have been suggested to be located in the reactive site loop sequence and even in the whole P15–P1 sequence [78] and around amino acids 446–449 and 452–455 [79]. Presumably, these autoantibodies interfere with insertion of the loop into the central β-sheet. This concept is supported by the suggestion that the sequence 452–455 is also involved in a secondary C1s binding site [20].

Summary

C1-INH belongs to the family of serpins. Structural studies have yielded a clear understanding of the biochemical principle underlying the functional activities of these proteins. Although the crystal structure of C1-INH has yet to be revealed, homology modeling has provided a three-dimensional model of the serpin part of C1-INH. This model has helped us understand the biochemical consequences of mutations of the C1-INH gene as they occur in patients who have HAE. The structure of the N-terminal domain of C1-INH remains unknown; however, this part of the molecule is unlikely to be important in the inhibitory activity of C1-INH toward its target proteases. Mutations in this part have not been described in patients who have HAE, except for a deletion containing two cysteine residues involved in the stabilization of the serpin domain. Recent studies suggest some anti-inflammatory functions for this N-terminal part, possibly explaining the effects of C1-INH in diseases other than HAE.

References

[1] Donaldson VH, Evans RR. A biochemical abnormality in hereditary angioneurotic edema. Am J Med 1963;35:37–44.
[2] Landermann NS, Webster ME, Becker EL, et al. Hereditary angioneurotic edema. II. Deficiency of inhibitor for serum globulin permeability factor and/or plasma kallikrein. Allergy 1962;33:330–41.

[3] Komiyama T, Ray CA, Pickup DJ, et al. Inhibition of interleukin-1 beta converting enzyme by the cowpox virus serpin CrmA. An example of cross-class inhibition. J Biol Chem 1994; 269(30):19331–7.

[4] Elliott PR, Abrahams JP, Lomas DA. Wild-type alpha 1–antitrypsin is in the canonical inhibitory conformation. J Mol Biol 1998;275(3):419–25.

[5] Li J, Wang Z, Canagarajah B, et al. The structure of active serpin 1K from Manduca sexta. Structure 1999;7(1):103–9.

[6] Stein PE, Leslie AG, Finch JT, et al. Crystal structure of uncleaved ovalbumin at 1.95 A resolution. J Mol Biol 1991;221(3):941–59.

[7] Skinner R, Abrahams JP, Whisstock JC, et al. The 2.6 A structure of antithrombin indicates a conformational change at the heparin binding site. J Mol Biol 1997;266(3):601–9.

[8] Loebermann H, Tokuoka R, Deisenhofer J, et al. Human alpha 1–proteinase inhibitor. Crystal structure analysis of two crystal modifications, molecular model and preliminary analysis of the implications for function. J Mol Biol 1984;177(3):531–57.

[9] Huntington JA, Read RJ, Carrell RW. Structure of a serpin-protease complex shows inhibition by deformation. Nature 2000;407(6806):923–6.

[10] Stavridi ES, O'Malley K, Lukacs CM, et al. Structural change in alpha-chymotrypsin induced by complexation with alpha 1–antichymotrypsin as seen by enhanced sensitivity to proteolysis. Biochemistry 1996;35(33):10608–15.

[11] Dementiev A, Dobo J, Gettins PG. Active site distortion is sufficient for proteinase inhibition by serpins: structure of the covalent complex of alpha1–proteinase inhibitor with porcine pancreatic elastase. J Biol Chem 2006;281(6):3452–7.

[12] Patston PA, Gettins P, Beechem J, et al. Mechanism of serpin action: evidence that C1 inhibitor functions as a suicide substrate. Biochemistry 1991;30(36):8876–82.

[13] Brown EW, Ravindran S, Patston PA. The reaction between plasmin and C1-inhibitor results in plasmin inhibition by the serpin mechanism. Blood Coagul Fibrinolysis 2002;13(8):711–4.

[14] Whisstock J, Skinner R, Lesk AM. An atlas of serpin conformations. Trends Biochem Sci 1998;23(2):63–7.

[15] Carrell RW. How serpins are shaping up. Science 1999;285(5435):1861.

[16] Gettins PG. Serpin structure, mechanism, and function. Chem Rev 2002;102(12):4751–804.

[17] Bock SC, Skriver K, Nielsen E, et al. Human C1 inhibitor: primary structure, cDNA cloning, and chromosomal localization. Biochemistry 1986;25(15):4292–301.

[18] Bos IG, Hack CE, Abrahams JP. Structural and functional aspects of C1-inhibitor. Immunobiology 2002;205(4–5):518–33.

[19] Bos IG, Lubbers YT, Eldering E, et al. Effect of reactive site loop elongation on the inhibitory activity of C1-inhibitor. Biochim Biophys Acta 2004;1699(1–2):139–44.

[20] He S, Sim RB, Whaley K. A secondary C1s interaction site on C1-inhibitor is essential for formation of a stable enzyme-inhibitor complex. FEBS Lett 1997;405(1):42–6.

[21] Bos IG, Lubbers YT, Roem D, et al. The functional integrity of the serpin domain of C1-inhibitor depends on the unique N-terminal domain, as revealed by a pathological mutant. J Biol Chem 2003;278(32):29463–70.

[22] Pixley RA, Schapira M, Colman RW. The regulation of human factor XIIa by plasma proteinase inhibitors. J Biol Chem 1985;260(3):1723–9.

[23] Chan JY, Burrowes CE, Habal FM, et al. The inhibition of activated factor XII (Hageman factor) by antithrombin III: the effect of other plasma proteinase inhibitors. Biochem Biophys Res Commun 1977;74(1):150–8.

[24] van der Graaf F, Koedam JA, Bouma BN. Inactivation of kallikrein in human plasma. J Clin Invest 1983;71(1):149–58.

[25] Schapira M, Scott CF, Colman RW. Contribution of plasma protease inhibitors to the inactivation of kallikrein in plasma. J Clin Invest 1982;69(2):462–8.

[26] Wuillemin WA, Minnema M, Meijers JC, et al. Inactivation of factor XIa in human plasma assessed by measuring factor XIa–protease inhibitor complexes: major role for C1-inhibitor. Blood 1995;85(6):1517–26.

[27] Sim RB, Reboul A, Arlaud GJ, et al. Interaction of 125I-labelled complement subcomponents C-1r and C-1s with protease inhibitors in plasma. FEBS Lett 1979;97(1):111–5.

[28] Schapira M, de Agostini A, Schifferli JA, et al. Biochemistry and pathophysiology of human C1 inhibitor: current issues. Complement 1985;2(2–3):111–26.

[29] Cooper NR. The classical complement pathway: activation and regulation of the first complement component. Adv Immunol 1985;37:151–216.

[30] Matsushita M, Thiel S, Jensenius JC, et al. Proteolytic activities of two types of mannose-binding lectin-associated serine protease. J Immunol 2000;165(5):2637–42.

[31] Skriver K, Radziejewska E, Silbermann JA, et al. CpG mutations in the reactive site of human C1 inhibitor. J Biol Chem 1989;264(6):3066–71.

[32] Zahedi R, Wisnieski J, Davis AE. Role of the P2 residue of complement 1 inhibitor (Ala443) in determination of target protease specificity: inhibition of complement and contact system proteases. J Immunol 1997;159(2):983–8.

[33] Zahedi R, Bissler JJ, Davis AE, et al. Unique C1 inhibitor dysfunction in a kindred without angioedema. II. Identification of an Ala443 → Val substitution and functional analysis of the recombinant mutant protein. J Clin Invest 1995;95(3):1299–305.

[34] Zahedi R, MacFarlane RC, Wisnieski JJ, et al. C1 inhibitor: analysis of the role of amino acid residues within the reactive center loop in target protease recognition. J Immunol 2001;167(3):1500–6.

[35] Eldering E, Huijbregts CC, Lubbers YT, et al. Characterization of recombinant C1 inhibitor P1 variants. J Biol Chem 1992;267(10):7013–20.

[36] Cugno M, Bos I, Lubbers Y, et al. In vitro interaction of C1-inhibitor with thrombin. Blood Coagul Fibrinolysis 2001;12(4):253–60.

[37] Jiang H, Wagner E, Zhang H, et al. Complement 1 inhibitor is a regulator of the alternative complement pathway. J Exp Med 2001;194(11):1609–16.

[38] Davis AE, Aulak K, Parad RB, et al. C1 inhibitor hinge region mutations produce dysfunction by different mechanisms. Nat Genet 1992;1(5):354–8.

[39] Davis AE. C1 inhibitor. Functional analysis of naturally-occurring mutant proteins. Adv Exp Med Biol 1997;425:185–94.

[40] Bos IG, de Bruin EC, Karuntu YA, et al. Recombinant human C1-inhibitor produced in Pichia pastoris has the same inhibitory capacity as plasma C1-inhibitor. Biochim Biophys Acta 2003;1648(1–2):75–83.

[41] Tenner AJ, Frank MM. Activator-bound C1 is less susceptible to inactivation by C1 inhibition than is fluid-phase C1. J Immunol 1986;137(2):625–30.

[42] Doekes G, van Es LA, Daha MR. C1-inactivator: its efficiency as a regulator of classical complement pathway activation by soluble IgG aggregates. Immunology 1983;49(2):215–22.

[43] Wuillemin WA, te Velthuis H, Lubbers YT, et al. Potentiation of C1 inhibitor by glycosaminoglycans: dextran sulfate species are effective inhibitors of in vitro complement activation in plasma. J Immunol 1997;159(4):1953–60.

[44] Wuillemin WA, Eldering E, Citarella F, et al. Modulation of contact system proteases by glycosaminoglycans. Selective enhancement of the inhibition of factor XIa. J Biol Chem 1996; 271(22):12913–8.

[45] Gozzo AJ, Nunes VA, Nader HB, et al. Glycosaminoglycans affect the interaction of human plasma kallikrein with plasminogen, factor XII and inhibitors. Braz J Med Biol Res 2003; 36(8):1055–9.

[46] Lathem WW, Bergsbaken T, Welch RA. Potentiation of C1 esterase inhibitor by StcE, a metalloprotease secreted by Escherichia coli O157:H7. J Exp Med 2004;199(8):1077–87.

[47] Black SC, Gralinski MR, Friedrichs GS, et al. Cardioprotective effects of heparin or N-acetylheparin in an in vivo model of myocardial ischaemic and reperfusion injury. Cardiovasc Res 1995;29(5):629–36.

[48] Friedrichs GS, Kilgore KS, Manley PJ, et al. Effects of heparin and N-acetyl heparin on ischemia/reperfusion–induced alterations in myocardial function in the rabbit isolated heart. Circ Res 1994;75(4):701–10.

[49] Weiler JM, Quinn SA, Woodworth GG, et al. Does heparin prophylaxis prevent exacerbations of hereditary angioedema? J Allergy Clin Immunol 2002;109(6):995–1000.

[50] Parish CR. Heparan sulfate and inflammation. Nat Immunol 2005;6(9):861–2.

[51] Coutinho M, Aulak KS, Davis AE. Functional analysis of the serpin domain of C1 inhibitor. J Immunol 1994;153(8):3648–54.

[52] Ravindran S, Grys TE, Welch RA, et al. Inhibition of plasma kallikrein by C1-inhibitor: role of endothelial cells and the amino-terminal domain of C1-inhibitor. Thromb Haemost 2004; 92(6):1277–83.

[53] Liu D, Cai S, Gu X, et al. C1 inhibitor prevents endotoxin shock via a direct interaction with lipopolysaccharide. J Immunol 2003;171(5):2594–601.

[54] Liu D, Cramer CC, Scafidi J, et al. N-linked glycosylation at Asn3 and the positively charged residues within the amino-terminal domain of the C1 inhibitor are required for interaction of the C1 inhibitor with Salmonella enterica serovar typhimurium lipopolysaccharide and lipid A. Infect Immun 2005;73(8):4478–87.

[55] Minta JO. The role of sialic acid in the functional activity and the hepatic clearance of C1-INH. J Immunol 1981;126(1):245–9.

[56] Reboul A, Prandini MH, Colomb MG. Proteolysis and deglycosylation of human C1 inhibitor. Effect on functional properties. Biochem J 1987;244(1):117–21.

[57] van Doorn MB, Burggraaf J, van Dam T, et al. A phase I study of recombinant human C1 inhibitor in asymptomatic patients with hereditary angioedema. J Allergy Clin Immunol 2005;116(4):876–83.

[58] Zhang F, Bries AD, Lang SC, et al. Metabolic alteration of the N-glycan structure of a protein from patients with a heterozygous protein deficiency. Biochim Biophys Acta 2004; 1739(1):43–9.

[59] De Graaf TW, Van der Stelt ME, Anbergen MG, et al. Inflammation-induced expression of sialyl Lewis X-containing glycan structures on alpha 1–acid glycoprotein (orosomucoid) in human sera. J Exp Med 1993;177(3):657–66.

[60] Brinkman–van der Linden EC, de Haan PF, Havenaar EC, et al. Inflammation-induced expression of sialyl LewisX is not restricted to alpha1-acid glycoprotein but also occurs to a lesser extent on alpha1-antichymotrypsin and haptoglobin. Glycoconj J 1998;15(2):177–82.

[61] Cai S, Davis AE III. Complement regulatory protein C1 inhibitor binds to selectins and interferes with endothelial-leukocyte adhesion. J Immunol 2003;171(9):4786–91.

[62] Cooper DN, Ball EV, Stensen PD, et al. The human gene mutation database at the Institute of Medical Genetics in Cardiff. Cardiff University 2006. Available at: http://www.hgmd.cf. ac.uk/. Accessed September 27, 2006.

[63] Kalmár L, Hegedûs T, Tordai A. The HAE Database. Available at: http://www.biomembrane. hu/hae/. Accessed September 27, 2006.

[64] Eldering E, Huijbregts CC, Nuijens JH, et al. Recombinant C1 inhibitor P5/P3 variants display resistance to catalytic inactivation by stimulated neutrophils. J Clin Invest 1993;91(3): 1035–43.

[65] Blanch A, Roche O, Lopez-Granados E, et al. Detection of C1 inhibitor (SERPING1/ C1NH) mutations in exon 8 in patients with hereditary angioedema: evidence for 10 novel mutations. Hum Mutat 2002;20(5):405–6.

[66] Aulak KS, Cicardi M, Harrison RA. Identification of a new P1 residue mutation (444Arg→ Ser) in a dysfunctional C1 inhibitor protein contained in a type II hereditary angioedema plasma. FEBS Lett 1990;266(1–2):13–6.

[67] Frangi D, Aulak KS, Cicardi M, et al. A dysfunctional C1 inhibitor protein with a new reactive center mutation (Arg-444→Leu). FEBS Lett 1992;301(1):34–6.

[68] Zahedi R, Aulak KS, Eldering E, et al. Characterization of C1 inhibitor-Ta. A dysfunctional C1INH with deletion of lysine 251. J Biol Chem 1996;271(39):24307–12.

[69] Aulak KS, Eldering E, Hack CE, et al. A hinge region mutation in C1-inhibitor (Ala436→ Thr) results in nonsubstrate-like behavior and in polymerization of the molecule. J Biol Chem 1993;268(24):18088–94.

[70] Verpy E, Couture-Tosi E, Eldering E, et al. Crucial residues in the carboxy-terminal end of C1 inhibitor revealed by pathogenic mutants impaired in secretion or function. J Clin Invest 1995;95(1):350–9.

[71] Eldering E, Verpy E, Roem D, et al. COOH-terminal substitutions in the serpin C1 inhibitor that cause loop overinsertion and subsequent multimerization. J Biol Chem 1995;270(6): 2579–87.

[72] Bowen B, Hawk JJ, Sibunka S, et al. A review of the reported defects in the human C1 esterase inhibitor gene producing hereditary angioedema including four new mutations. Clin Immunol 2001;98(2):157–63.

[73] Zuraw BL, Curd JG. Demonstration of modified inactive first component of complement (C1) inhibitor in the plasmas of C1 inhibitor–deficient patients. J Clin Invest 1986;78(2): 567–75.

[74] Malbran A, Hammer CH, Frank MM, et al. Acquired angioedema: observations on the mechanism of action of autoantibodies directed against C1 esterase inhibitor. J Allergy Clin Immunol 1988;81(6):1199–204.

[75] Jackson J, Sim RB, Whelan A, et al. An IgG autoantibody which inactivates C1-inhibitor. Nature 1986;323(6090):722–4.

[76] Jackson J, Sim RB, Whaley K, et al. Autoantibody facilitated cleavage of C1-inhibitor in autoimmune angioedema. J Clin Invest 1989;83(2):698–707.

[77] Alsenz J, Lambris JD, Bork K, et al. Acquired C1 inhibitor (C1-INH) deficiency type II. Replacement therapy with C1-INH and analysis of patients' C1-INH and anti–C1-INH autoantibodies. J Clin Invest 1989;83(6):1794–9.

[78] Mandle R, Baron C, Roux E, et al. Acquired C1 inhibitor deficiency as a result of an autoantibody to the reactive center region of C1 inhibitor. J Immunol 1994;152(9):4680–5.

[79] He S, Tsang S, North J, et al. Epitope mapping of C1 inhibitor autoantibodies from patients with acquired C1 inhibitor deficiency. J Immunol 1996;156(5):2009–13.

ELSEVIER
SAUNDERS

Immunol Allergy Clin N Am
26 (2006) 633–651

IMMUNOLOGY
AND ALLERGY
CLINICS
OF NORTH AMERICA

Mechanism of Angioedema in First Complement Component Inhibitor Deficiency

Alvin E. Davis III, MD

CBR Institute for Biomedical Research, Harvard Medical School,
800 Huntington Avenue, Boston, MA 02115, USA

Characterization of the pathophysiology of hereditary angioedema (HAE) began in 1962 with the observation by Landerman and colleagues [1] that plasma of patients who had hereditary angioedema was deficient in plasma kallikrein inhibitory capacity and the subsequent demonstration by Donaldson and Evans [2] that the deficient protein was first complement component (C1) inhibitor. The role of C1 inhibitor in regulation of complement system activation had been described shortly after the first description of the isolation and characterization of the first complement component; it was characterized as a heat labile factor in plasma that inhibited the esterolytic activity of C1 [3]. C1 was shown to consist of three separate proteins, C1q, C1r, and C1s, the last two of which are zymogen serine proteases that are converted to their proteolytically active forms following binding of C1q to an immune complex. Subsequent studies demonstrated that C1 inhibitor inactivates both C1r and C1s [4,5].

The role of C1 inhibitor in regulation of the contact system, by means of inactivation of both plasma kallikrein and factor XIIa, was elucidated during the 1970s and 1980s [6–14]. C1 inhibitor also is capable of inactivating a number of other proteases, including plasmin and tissue plasminogen activator (tPA) [15–19]. The evidence clearly indicates that C1 inhibitor is not a major regulator of plasmin, which, in vivo, is inhibited primarily by α_2 antiplasmin [20,21]. Some data, however, suggest that C1 inhibitor may participate in tPA inactivation [16]. Cugno and colleagues [22,23] have demonstrated activation of both the coagulation cascade and the fibrinolytic

Many of the studies described here were supported by USPHS grants HD22082, HD33727, and AI057366.

E-mail address: aldavis@cbrinstitute.org

doi:10.1016/j.iac.2006.08.003   *immunology.theclinics.com*

pathway during attacks of HAE. Therefore, C1 inhibitor may be involved in regulation of these pathways in vivo or, alternatively, activation of these pathways by exogenous factors may trigger attacks of angioedema.

One might have expected that the demonstration of the specific deficiency responsible for HAE and characterization of the proteases inactivated by C1 inhibitor would lead rapidly to characterization of the mechanism of generation of angioedema symptoms. However, largely because C1 inhibitor is the primary regulator of activation of both the classic pathway of complement and the contact system of kinin generation, the mechanism remained unclear until recently. At this point, the accumulated information clearly indicates that the primary, and most likely the sole, mediator of symptoms is bradykinin generated by means of activation of the contact system. However, the specific biochemical events leading to the initiation of an angioedema attack remain ill defined.

Function of first complement component inhibitor

C1 inhibitor is a member of the serpins, a family of proteins consisting mostly, but not solely, of serine protease inhibitors. All members of the serpin family share similar sequences and three-dimensional structures and consist of seven to nine α helices and three β sheets. The most distinctive features of the native serpin structure are a five-stranded β sheet (sheet A) that makes up the prominent planar surface of the molecule and a peptide loop (the reactive center loop) consisting of approximately 17 amino acid residues that is exposed at one pole of the molecule. The reactive center loop is located near the carboxyl terminus of the protein. The native serpin structure is rather unstable and is sensitive to denaturing conditions. Cleavage by a nontarget protease within the reactive center loop results in a dramatic molecular rearrangement, with insertion of this loop into β sheet A as its fourth strand, converting sheet A to a six-stranded sheet. The cleaved inhibitor is a much more stable structure that may be demonstrated by enhanced resistance to thermal or chemical denaturation [24–26]. This rearrangement is indicated by the expression of neoepitopes on the cleaved molecule [27–29].

Serpins inactivate proteases after recognition by the protease of a substrate-like sequence located within the reactive center loop. The protease attacks the peptide bond carboxyl terminal to the P1 residue, which, in the case of C1 inhibitor, is an arginine. The inhibitor is cleaved at this site. However, rather than subsequent release of the protease, a covalent bond is formed between the reactive center amino acid residue of the serpin and the active site serine of the protease [30]. Subsequently, the reactive center loop inserts into β sheet A, as with cleavage by nontarget proteases. This insertion moves the protease to the opposite pole of the molecule. The result is a stable cleaved serpin structure covalently linked to a destabilized protease in which its catalytic triad is interrupted. Both the protease and the inhibitor are thereby inactivated, an aspect that led to the designation of serpins as suicide substrates [31]. The structural and functional data all indicate that the mechanism of inactivation of proteases by C1 inhibitor is the same as the mechanism with other serpins [31,32].

The most significant difference between C1 inhibitor and other serpins is in the size and characteristics of its nonserpin amino terminal domain. This domain in C1 inhibitor is quite large (approximately 100 residues) and is heavily glycosylated with three N-linked and at least seven O-linked carbohydrates [33]. Some portions of the sequence of this domain are mucin-like. Based on functional studies using a recombinant C1 inhibitor molecule with the amino terminal 100 residues deleted, this domain plays no role in protease inhibitor function [34]. Recent studies have indicated that the amino terminal domain is required, however, for a direct interaction with gram-negative bacteria and endotoxins [35,36]. This interaction may play a role in C1 inhibitor–mediated protection from sepsis and septic shock.

C1 inhibitor is the only protease inhibitor that inactivates C1r and C1s [4,5] and is, therefore, the primary regulator of classic pathway activation (Fig. 1). It also plays a role in regulation of the lectin pathway, which is activated by interaction of mannan-binding lectin or ficolins with surface structures of a variety of micro-organisms [37–39]. C1 inhibitor inactivates MASP2, a C1s-like protease that is associated with mannan binding lectin and ficolins and is activated following binding. However, in vivo, MASP2 also most likely is inactivated by α_2 macroglobulin [40]. The relative importance of each is not yet clear. Another complement regulatory function of C1 inhibitor has been described, in which C1 inhibitor was shown to bind to C3b, which resulted in inhibition of factor B binding, similar to the mechanism of action of factor H [41]. This function was independent of protease inhibitor activity. Although the resulting alternative pathway inhibition was shown to take place at physiologic concentrations in vitro, the importance of this activity in vivo remains unclear.

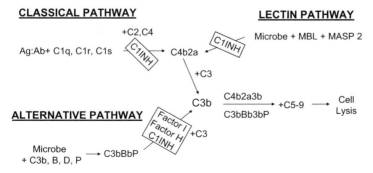

Fig. 1. Complement system activation. The components enclosed within rectangles are inhibitors of activation. Ag:Ab, antigen-antibody complexes; B, factor B; C1INH, C1 inhibitor; D, factor D; MASP 2, Mannan-binding lectin associated protease 2; MBL, mannan-binding lectin; P, properdin.

C1 inhibitor is the primary inhibitor of both plasma kallikrein and coagulation factor XIIa, although these proteases can also be inactivated by α_2 macroglobulin [6,9,12–14]. It is therefore the major regulator of contact system–mediated bradykinin generation. By virtue of its inactivaton of both factor XIIa and factor XIa, C1 inhibitor also inhibits activation of the intrinsic coagulation pathway. The contact system is activated by a variety of exogenous negatively charged surfaces, such as glass, kaolin, elagic acid, dextran sulfate, and possibly endotoxin lipopolysaccharide [42–47]. Factor XII binds to these surfaces; this binding induces its autoactivation to proteolytically active factor XIIa, which activates both plasma prekallikrein and additional factor XII (Fig. 2). Activated kallikrein then cleaves two peptide bonds in high molecular weight kininogen to release bradykinin. A biologically relevant negatively charged substance responsible for activation in vivo has not been described. Activation in vivo most likely takes place primarily on the surface of endothelial cells [48–53].

At least two pathways that lead to activation of kallikrein in the absence of factor XII have been described. One of these is reported to be mediated by an interaction between the kallikrein–high molecular weight kininogen complex and heat shock protein 90 [50,54,55], whereas the other depends on activation of prekallikrein by prolylcarboxypeptidase (see Fig. 2) [56–59]. Some data suggest that the prolylcarboxypeptidase-mediated activation mechanism is quite efficient and may be the primary mechanism of contact system activation in vivo [56,59]. By contrast, other data suggest that both this and heat shock protein 90–mediated activation are quite slow, but that they are greatly accelerated in the presence of factor XII [50,54,55]. Although the details of contact system activation remain to be resolved, it is

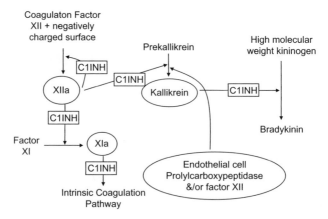

Fig. 2. Contact system activation. The diagram indicates the two pathways of contact system activation, one by means of exogenous negatively charged surfaces and the other taking place on the surface of endothelial cells. Activation of prekallikrein on endothelial cells is proposed to be mediated by prolylcarboxypeptidase or by factor XII. C1INH, C1 inhibitor.

clear that the primary mechanism of regulation of activation of the contact system is inhibition of kallikrein (and factor XIIa) by C1 inhibitor.

Mutations resulting in first complement component inhibitor deficiency

Individuals who have HAE are heterozygous for mutations that result either in lack of expression of C1 inhibitor protein or in the synthesis of a nonfunctional protein from one allele together with expression of normal protein from the other allele. Clinically, these two types are referred to as type 1 and type 2, respectively, based on whether a dysfunctional protein is detectable in the patient's plasma. However, this division is not precisely accurate. A number of mutations result in a dysfunctional protein that is either degraded intracellularly, secreted inefficiently, or cleared rapidly from the circulation. Strictly speaking, these should be referred to as type 2, but, because they are either absent or present in very small quantities in the blood, they are usually classified as type 1. In clinical practice, a patient is classified as type 2 based on the finding of a normal (or elevated) C1 inhibitor level determined immunochemically, together with a decreased functional level of C1 inhibitor. Using these criteria, approximately 80% to 85% of patients are classified as type 1.

Mutations resulting in deficiency may be of virtually any type, including deletions (and duplications) that range in size from a few base pairs to multiple exons and a variety of single base substitutions. Large deletions and single base changes at the reactive center are somewhat overrepresented in comparison with the other types of mutations. All of the large mutations appear to be a consequence of recombination involving the multiple Alu repetitive elements that are present within the introns of the gene. The reactive center mutations most likely are a result of the cytosine-guanine (CG) dinucleotide within the codon for the reactive center arginine (CGC). The CG dinucleotide is susceptible to mutation due to deamidation of methylated cytosine, which results in conversion to a thymine. This process may occur in the CG dinucleotide in the coding strand or in the complementary strand. With C1 inhibitor, this results in substitution of the reactive center arginine with either cysteine or histidine. These make up the largest single group of mutations within the C1 inhibitor gene. However, it should be noted that some other mechanism may also be at play here, because several serine and leucine substitutions at the reactive center have been described, which cannot result from the deamidation mechanism.

Whether a patient is type 1 or type 2 is of no known clinical importance. No differences exist between the two in clinical presentation, severity, or clinical course. Furthermore, with two possible exceptions, the specific mutation does not appear to have any clinical effect. These potential exceptions are one family with a large deletion, in which the abnormal transcript appears to inhibit transcription of the normal gene, and another family with a small duplication, which appears to result in inhibition of translation of the normal C1 inhibitor transcript [60,61]. It is not known whether these mechanisms apply in other families with different mutations.

Pathophysiologic interpretation of clinical characteristics

Patients who have HAE develop recurrent acute episodes of localized edema that may involve the skin, the mucosa of the gastrointestinal tract, the pharynx, or the larynx. Therefore, patients who have C1 inhibitor deficiency have an intermittent defect in the regulation of vascular permeability. This increased vascular permeability results from a sudden local loss of endothelial barrier function within the postcapillary venule. Signs or symptoms of inflammation are absent, as are any signs of an allergic component. Although early reports suggested that urinary histamine levels were elevated during attacks of angioedema, antihistamines are ineffective, and a study of a number of patients who had HAE (both symptomatic and asymptomatic) demonstrated that urinary histamine levels are not elevated [62]. The angioedema in HAE does not respond to treatment with epinephrine.

Serpins are suicide substrates, which may be one important factor in the initiation of attacks of angioedema. Activation of any protease inhibited by C1 inhibitor, whether a complement, contact, or fibrinolytic system protease, will result in inactivation and consumption of the inhibitor. If the rate of consumption exceeds the rate of ongoing synthesis, the C1 inhibitor plasma level will decrease. C1 inhibitor levels in patients who have HAE average approximately 30% of normal during symptom-free periods. Significant reduction below this level is associated with the development of symptoms. Therefore, any event that triggers activation of any of the three proteolytic pathways would increase C1 inhibitor consumption and suppress the plasma level and could result in an episode of angioedema. Clearly, trauma and inflammation, which are known initiators of attacks of angioedema, can result in activation of each pathway. However, not all episodes of angioedema are associated with an obvious precipitating factor. In addition, consumption of C1 inhibitor could be amplified if activation of one system directly resulted in activation of either or both of the other two systems (Fig. 3). Activated factor XII and plasmin may activate C1, and factor XIIa or kallikrein may generate plasmin from plasminogen, but the biologic significance of these findings has not been clearly demonstrated [63–69].

Another possibility with some clinical support is that plasmin generation might activate the contact system, with resulting bradykinin generation, and might thus result in the development of angioedema. Angioedema sometimes develops during therapy with recombinant tissue plasminogen activator [70,71]. Experimental evidence suggests that this angioedema is mediated by bradykinin released by the plasmin that is generated by the infused tissue plasminogen activator [71,72]. It is possible that, in a patient who has HAE, activation of the fibrinolytic pathway during trauma or inflammation might generate sufficient plasmin for a similar phenomenon to occur.

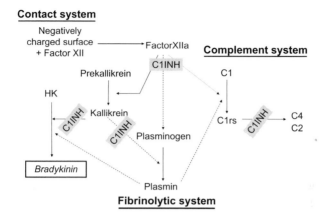

Fig. 3. Proposed interactions among the complement, contact, and fibrinolytic systems. Arrows with solid lines indicate reactions of known biologic relevance. Arrows with dotted lines indicate reactions demonstrated to take place in vitro, but that are of uncertain in vivo importance. C1INH, C1 inhibitor; HK, high molecular weight kininogen.

This hypothesis is consistent with the clinical observation that plasmin inhibitors are frequently effective in HAE.

The mediation of angioedema

Complement system activation

In HAE, the low plasma levels of C1 inhibitor result in apparent spontaneous activation of both the complement and contact systems. Although this is most obvious during an overt attack of angioedema, it is highly likely that activation occurs to some degree during symptom-free periods. C2 and C4 levels, which are virtually always low during an attack, may also be low when the patient is asymptomatic [73–75]. Another indication of activation is the observation that the catabolic rate of C1 inhibitor in symptom-free HAE patients is elevated in comparison with that of normal individuals [76]. This aspect also probably accounts for the finding that plasma levels of C1 inhibitor are much less than 50% of normal, which would be expected in a heterozygous deficiency state [77]. During periods of angioedema, circulating activated C1 [73,78] and complexes of C1 inhibitor with both C1r and C1s may be detected [79], in addition to decreased plasma levels of C2 and C4, which may be so low as to be undetectable.

During the 1970s and 1980s, a number of studies were published that suggested that the mediator of angioedema was a product of complement system activation. On a clinical basis, a complement-derived mediator appeared most likely to many investigators because angioedema is nonpainful, whereas subcutaneous injection of bradykinin, which also produces edema, is quite painful. Donaldson and colleagues [80] showed that plasma taken from

HAE patients during symptom-free periods, following incubation at 37°C, generated a factor that contracted smooth muscle and had vascular permeability–enhancing activity when it was injected intradermally into guinea pig skin. The data suggested that this kinin-like activity was derived from complement activation; furthermore, both C2 and C4 appeared to be required for its generation [80–82]. Specifically, the factor appeared to differ from bradykinin in size, electrophoretic mobility, isoelectric point, and susceptibility to trypsin, and its generation was inhibited by antibodies to C2 and C4.

Various other data also appeared to support the hypothesis that the mediator was complement derived. Intradermal injection, in guinea pigs and humans, of proteolytically active C1s resulted in local swelling without pain or itching (ie, it was similar to angioedema) [83–85]. Furthermore, C2-deficient people did not respond to intradermal injection of C1s, whereas a C3-deficient patient did respond [84,86]. C2-deficient guinea pigs also were unresponsive, but the response was restored following intravenous infusion of C2 [87]. Therefore, to induce a vascular permeability response by means of complement activation, C2 was required. However, these studies did not identify the source of the mediator. In addition, there were no clearcut direct data to indicate that the mediator resulting from complement system activation was the same as the mediator responsible for angioedema in HAE.

Several studies suggested that the complement-derived factor might result from plasmin cleavage of C2 during complement activation. First, mixtures of C1s, C2, and plasmin, in the presence or absence of C4, generated vascular permeability–enhancing and smooth muscle–contracting activity [88,89]. This event appeared to coincide with the release of a group of small peptides from the carboxyl terminus of C2b [88]. In addition, several synthetic peptides matching the carboxyl terminal sequence of C2b possessed vascular permeability and smooth muscle–contracting activity [88]. The most active of these was 25 amino acids long. However, although this synthetic peptide clearly enhanced vascular permeability, its specific activity was low in comparison with bradykinin. Another study was unable to demonstrate any cleavage of C2 or C2b with plasmin, and no kinin-like activity resulted from such incubation mixtures [90].

Contact system activation

During the same period, evidence for contact system activation in HAE was also accumulating. Among the first of these findings was the demonstration that large amounts of active kallikrein were present in induced blister fluid from patients who had HAE. This finding suggested a lower threshold for contact system activation in comparison with normal individuals [91]. In addition, during attacks, patients who had HAE had decreased levels of prekallikrein and of high molecular weight kininogen [92]. At least two early studies suggested that bradykinin was generated during attacks of angioedema [93,94]. One of these reported, unfortunately only in abstract form, that bradykinin was directly detectable in plasma from HAE patients following in vitro incubation [93]. In 1986, Berrettini and colleagues [95] demonstrated that high molecular weight kininogen was circulating in a cleaved form in a patient who had HAE. Subsequently, this group and a number of others have confirmed this finding in additional patients [96–99].

Therefore, by the end of the 1980s, it was clear that both the complement and contact systems were activated during episodes of angioedema. However, the precise mediator in HAE had not been unequivocally identified. Many investigators believed that the mediator was bradykinin, whereas others believed that a "C2 kinin" was responsible. In 1994, Shoemaker and colleagues [100] sought to begin to clarify this issue by repeating, as closely as possible, the protocol followed previously by Donaldson and colleagues [80]. For these experiments, in addition to HAE plasma, "artificial HAE plasma" was prepared by immunoabsorption with anti–C1 inhibitor antibody. This technique made possible the use of a variety of deficient plasmas, which then also were made deficient in C1 inhibitor. Vascular permeability–enhancing activity could be generated both from HAE remission plasma and from normal plasma depleted of C1 inhibitor. More importantly, the activity was also readily generated from C1 inhibitor–depleted C2-deficient plasma, but not from plasma deficient in prekallikrein, factor XII, or high molecular weight kininogen. Furthermore, the active factor was isolated and shown by amino acid sequence analysis to be bradykinin [100]. Subsequently, Nussberger and colleagues [101] demonstrated that bradykinin levels were elevated in the plasmas of patients who had HAE during episodes of angioedema. Although these data do not demonstrate a cause and effect relationship between bradykinin and angioedema, they strongly suggest that bradykinin is involved. The data also do not rule out the possibility that more than one mediator is involved.

A dysfunctional first complement component inhibitor
with diminished inhibition of complement proteases
but normal inhibition of contact system proteases

In 1994, Wisnieski and colleagues [102] described a kindred with extremely low C4 levels as a result of an apparent dysfunctional C1 inhibitor molecule that was defective in its capacity to inhibit C1. This defect presumably resulted in excessive C4 consumption. The propositus from this family presented with systemic lupus erythematosus. Subsequent studies demonstrated that every family member with a low C4 level expressed a C1 inhibitor molecule that was defective in its ability to inhibit both C1r and C1s but retained a perfectly normal ability to inactivate plasma kallikrein and coagulation factor XII [103–105]. This mutant C1 inhibitor retained only approximately 10% of its ability to inhibit proteolytically active C1r and C1s. This dysfunction was due to a mutation that resulted in substitution of the alanine residue immediately amino terminal to the reactive center arginine (the P2 position, Ala443) with a valine [103]. Most importantly, neither the single patient who has systemic lupus nor any of the seven other family members who express this dysfunctional protein has ever had angioedema. These individuals clearly had ongoing complement system activation, as indicated by their depressed plasma C4 levels. Therefore, complement system activation alone does not result in the generation of any peptide that induces angioedema. This family provides strong indirect evidence that the mediator in HAE is bradykinin.

The first complement component inhibitor–deficient mouse

Analysis of C1 inhibitor knockout mice has provided additional support for the hypothesis that bradykinin is the mediator of angioedema in HAE [106]. A database of genes randomly targeted with a retroviral-mediated gene trapping technique developed by Lexicon Genetics (The Woodlands, Texas) was screened. The C1 inhibitor gene was targeted in two embryonic stem cell lines, one of which was used to develop the deficient mice. Both the C1 inhibitor heterozygous deficient (C1INH$^{+/-}$) and homozyous deficient (C1INH$^{-/-}$) mice were normal in appearance, grew and developed normally, and reproduced normally. Litter size was normal in both C1INH$^{+/-}$ and C1INH$^{-/-}$ matings, which suggests that there was no increase in embryonic or fetal death. Neither C1 inhibitor mRNA nor protein was detected in C1INH$^{-/-}$ mice. Similar to observations in patients who have HAE, C1 inhibitor plasma levels in C1INH$^{+/-}$ mice were less than 50% of normal. C4 protein levels and functional complement levels were variably decreased in most C1 inhibitor–deficient mice, although probably not to such an extent as in humans who have HAE. Therefore, the mice appear to have unregulated complement activation, although possibly not to such an extent as do patients who have HAE.

Another indication that the consequences of C1-inhibitor deficiency in the mouse are less dramatic than in the human is provided by the observation that none of the mice have ever developed angioedema involving the skin. A total of only eight deficient mice have had spontaneous episodes of gastrointestinal edema with obstruction; one of these mice also had laryngeal edema. None of the wild-type littermate mice were affected, nor were any other mice in the colony. However, the episodes have not recurred in other deficient mice. Unfortunately, the trigger for these episodes is unknown, and attempts to reproduce such episodes have not been successful. Although these events did appear to be angioedema, it is not possible definitively to ascribe them to C1 inhibitor deficiency, both because they have not been reproduced and because no biochemical data exist from the time of the attacks.

Although C1 inhibitor–deficient mice do not have any clinically apparent abnormalities, when a marker for plasma protein extravasation (Evans Blue dye) was used, the mice were shown to have increased vascular permeability in comparison with wild-type littermate controls (C1INH$^{+/+}$). C1INH$^{-/-}$, C1INH$^{+/-}$, and C1INH$^{+/+}$ mice were injected intravenously with Evans blue dye, which readily binds to serum albumin. Within minutes, the skin of the feet and the skin around the nose and eyes of both the heterozygous and homozygous deficient mice became quite blue, whereas that of the wild-type mice became only slightly blue (Fig. 4) [106]. The vascular permeability was increased to a greater extent than in the wild-type mice by the topical application of mustard oil, which enhances local inflammation. The degree of vascular permeability was quantitated spectrophotometrically by extraction of the dye from the feet of the mice. The dye extravasation both in the C1INH$^{+/-}$ and in the C1INH$^{-/-}$ mice was approximately 1.5 times greater than that in the wild-type mice (Table 1). Enhancement with mustard oil increased the difference to 3- to 3.5-fold greater in the deficient mice. Treatment of the deficient mice with intravenous C1 inhibitor (100 µg) before injection with Evans blue dye completely reversed the increased vascular permeability. The amount of vascular leak in the treated deficient mice was indistinguishable from that of their wild-type littermates. This finding strongly indicates that the increase in vascular permeability in the knockout mice was solely a result of the deficiency of C1 inhibitor and not of some unexpected associated defect.

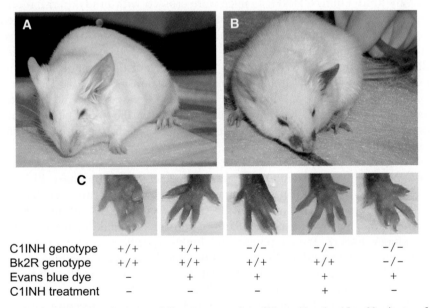

C1INH genotype	+/+	+/+	-/-	-/-	-/-
Bk2R genotype	+/+	+/+	+/+	+/+	-/-
Evans blue dye	-	+	+	+	+
C1INH treatment	-	-	-	+	-

Fig. 4. Analysis of vascular permeability. Extravasation of Evans blue dye 15 to 30 minutes after injection. (*A*) Wild-type mouse; (*B*) C1 inhibitor–deficient mouse; (*C*) rear footpads of mice of the indicated genotypes with or without C1 inhibitor treatment. Bk2R, bradykinin 2 receptor; C1INH, C1 inhibitor.

Table 1
Vascular permeability in C1-inhibitor-deficient mice

C1INH genotype	Bk2R genotype	No. of mice	C1INH treatment	Fold change in dye extravasation vs. WT[a]
+/−	+/+	5	None	1.5*
−/−	+/+	5	None	1.6*
−/−	−/−	5	None	1.0
+/−	+/+	4	C1INH	1.1
−/−	+/+	4	C1INH	1.0
−/−	+/+	22	DX-88	1.0
−/−	+/+	25	Icatibant	0.9
−/−	+/+	11	P2 A→V	1.0

Abbreviations: Bk2R, bradykinin 2 receptor; C1INH, C1 inhibitor; P2 A→V, P2 alanine to valine; WT, wild type.

[a] The dye extravasation was quantitated spectrophotometrically at 600 nm. The mean values of each group are expressed as the fold increase compared with an untreated wild-type control group.

* $P < .002$ compared with wild-type controls.

Data from Han ED, MacFarlane RC, Mulligan AN, et al. Increased vascular permeability in C1 inhibitor deficient mice is mediated by the bradykinin type 2 receptor. J Clin Invest 2002:109:1057–63; and Han Lee E, Pappalardo E, Scafidi J, et al. Approaches toward reversal of increased vascular permeability in C1 inhibitor deficient mice. Immuno Letters 2003;89:155–60.

To test the hypothesis that the increased vascular permeability was mediated by bradykinin, C1INH$^{-/-}$ mice were crossed with bradykinin 2 receptor (Bk2R) knockout mice. The resulting C1INH$^{+/-}$, Bk2R$^{+/-}$ mice then were mated, which resulted in all the expected genotypes in the predicted proportions. The C1INH$^{+/-}$, Bk2R$^{+/-}$ and the C1INH$^{-/-}$, Bk2R$^{-/-}$ mice all appeared normal. Furthermore, they were indistinguishable from the wild-type mice in their vascular permeability response (see Table 1). Therefore, the Bk2R is required to mediate the increased vascular permeability response. Bradykinin is the only known ligand for the Bk2R. These data strongly indicate that bradykinin is the mediator of the increased vascular permeability in the mice.

To confirm and strengthen these observations, mice also were treated with two agents that inhibit contact system activation but have little or no effect on complement system activation, and with another that is a Bk2R antagonist. The first agent, DX-88 (Dyax Corp., Cambridge, Massachusetts), is an engineered Kunitz domain protease inhibitor prepared using phage display. It is a potent and highly specific inhibitor of plasma kallikrein. The second kallikrein inhibitor used was the recombinant mutated C1 inhibitor in which the P2 Ala had been substituted with a Val [103–105], diminishing its inhibition of C1r and C1s but having no effect on its ability to inhibit plasma kallikrein. The bradykinin receptor antagonist used was Icatibant (Jerini AG, Berlin, Germany), a decapeptide antagonist with a structure similar to that of bradykinin. Each of these agents completely reversed the increased vascular permeability (see Table 1).

Because the bradykinin receptor antagonist and both inhibitors of contact system activation prevent the increased vascular permeability, it appears unlikely that any mediator other than bradykinin is involved.

Although the C1 inhibitor–deficient mice have an obvious defect in vascular permeability, they appear to have compensated quite well for this defect. Furthermore, it is surprising that the phenotype in these mice appears identical in the C1INH$^{+/-}$ and C1INH$^{-/-}$ mice. No human with complete deficiency of C1 inhibitor has been described, which suggests that complete deficiency might be lethal. The explanation for the relative mildness of the phenotype in the mice in comparison with humans who have angioedema is unknown, as is that for the lack of difference between the heterozygous and homozygous deficient mice. A likely potential explanation for both findings is that, in the mouse, other inhibitors play a larger role in regulation of C1 inhibitor target proteases than is the case in the human. For example, although in both the mouse and the human, C1 inhibitor appears to be the only inhibitor of activated C1r and C1s, in the human it is not the only inhibitor of factor XIIa and plasma kallikrein. Depending on the methods used, in human plasma C1 inhibitor provides from 42% to 84% of the kallikrein inhibitory capacity and as much as 90% of the inhibitory capacity toward activated factor XII [9,12–14,107]. The remainder of the plasma inhibitory activity toward both kallikrein and factor XIIa is provided by α_2 macroglobulin. It is possible that α_2 macroglobulin, or perhaps other inhibitors, provides a higher proportion of the inhibition of murine contact system proteases. This hypothesis remains uninvestigated.

Another potential explanation for the lack of difference between C1INH$^{+/-}$ and C1INH$^{-/-}$ mice is that, below a critical C1 inhibitor level, activation of the complement and contact systems is maximal, and a further decrease in the C1 inhibitor level has no additional effect. However, at least for the complement system, this is unlikely to be the case, because the C4 and hemolytic complement levels, although lower than in wild-type mice, are only moderately reduced. It also appears unlikely, therefore, that maximal activation of the contact system would occur. Another possibility is that the kallikrein substrate, high molecular weight kininogen, is depleted in both the C1INH$^{+/-}$ and C1INH$^{-/-}$ mice. The resolution of these questions awaits the development of appropriate reagents for these measurements.

The contributions of new therapeutic approaches toward definition of the pathophysiology of angioedema

Clinical trials using DX88 and Icatibant, the two new therapeutic agents described earlier, have provided further evidence supporting the hypothesis that angioedema in HAE is mediated by bradykinin. In the case of DX-88, two Phase II clinical trials have been completed, a third Phase II trial is nearly complete, and a Phase III trial is ongoing [108]. Icatibant has been used in one completed Phase II clinical trial, and two Phase III trials are currently ongoing [109]. From the available data, both agents appear to be quite effective, in that they decrease the time to beginning of symptom relief. Furthermore, at appropriate doses, they both appear to be effective in nearly all patients. The available results from these trials, therefore, confirm the conclusions from the experiments in the C1 inhibitor knockout mice and indicate clearly that the primary mediator of attacks of angioedema in humans is bradykinin.

References

[1] Landerman NS, Webster ME, Becker EL, et al. Hereditary angioneurotic edema. II. Deficiency of inhibitor for serum globulin permeability factor and/or plasma kallikrein. J Allergy 1962;33:330–41.
[2] Donaldson VH, Evans RR. A biochemical abnormality in hereditary angioneurotic edema. Am J Med 1963;35:37–44.
[3] Ratnoff O, Lepow I. Some properties of an esterase derived from preparations of the first component of complement. J Exp Med 1957;106:327–43.
[4] Sim RB, Reboul A, Arlaud GJ, et al. Interaction of 125I-labelled complement components C1r and C1s with protease inhibitors in plasma. FEBS Lett 1979;97:111–5.
[5] Ziccardi RJ. Activation of the early components of the classical complement pathway under physiological conditions. J Immunol 1981;126:1768–73.
[6] de Agostini A, Lijnen HR, Pixley RA, et al. Inactivation of factor-XII active fragment in normal plasma: predominant role of C1-inhibitor. J Clin Invest 1984;93:1542–9.
[7] Gallimore MJ, Amundsen E, Larsbraaten M, et al. Studies on plasma inhibitors of plasma kallikrein using chromogenic peptide substrate assays. Thromb Res 1979;16:695–703.
[8] Gigli I, Mason JW, Colman RW, et al. Interaction of plasma kallikrein with the C1 inhibitor. J Immunol 1970;104:574–81.
[9] Harpel PC, Lewin MF, Kaplan AP. Distribution of plasma kallikrein between C1 inactivator and a2-macroglobulin in plasma utilizing a new assay for a2-macroglobulin-kallikrein complexes. J Biol Chem 1985;260:4257–63.
[10] Lewin MF, Kaplan AP, Harpel PC. Studies of C1 inactivator–plasma kallikrein complexes in purified systems and in plasma. Quantitation by an enzyme-linked differential antibody immunosorbent assay. J Biol Chem 1983;258:6415–21.
[11] McConnell DJ. Inhibitors of kallikrein in human plasma. J Clin Invest 1972;51:1611–23.
[12] Pixley RA, Schapira M, Colman RW. The regulation of human factor XIIa by plasma proteinase inhibitors. J Biol Chem 1985;260:1723–9.
[13] Schapira M, Scott CF, Colman RW. Contribution of plasma protease inhibitors to the inactivation of kallikrein in plasma. J Clin Invest 1982;69:462–8.
[14] van der Graaf F, Koedam JA, Bouma BN. Inactivation of kallikrein in human plasma. J Clin Invest 1983;71:149–58.
[15] Harpel PC, Cooper NR. Studies on human plasma C1-inactivator-enzyme interactions. I. Mechanisms of interaction with C1s, plasmin and trypsin. J Clin Invest 1975;55: 593–604.
[16] Huisman LG, van Griensven JM, Kluft C. On the role of C1-inhibitor as inhibitor of tissue-type plasminogen activator in human plasma. Thromb Haemost 1995;73:466–71.
[17] Ranby M, Bergstorf N, Nilsson T. Enzymatic properties of one and two chain forms of tissue plasminogen activator. Thromb Res 1982;27:175–84.
[18] Ratnoff O, Pensky J, Ogston D, et al. The inhibition of plasmin, plasma kallikrein, plasma permeability factor, and the C1'r subcomponent of complement by serum C1' esterase inhibitor. J Exp Med 1969;129:315–31.

[19] Sulikowski T, Patston PA. The inhibition of TNK-t-PA by C1-inhibitor. Blood Coagul Fibrinolysis 2001;12:75–7.

[20] Aoki N, Moroi M, Matsuda M, et al. The behavior of alpha2-plasmin inhibitor in fibrinolytic states. J Clin Invest 1977;60:361–9.

[21] Harpel PC. Alpha2-plasmin inhibitor and alpha2-macroglobulin-plasmin complexes in plasma. Quantitation by an enzyme-linked differential antibody immunosorbent assay. J Clin Invest 1981;68:46–55.

[22] Cugno M, Cicardi M, Bottasso B, et al. Activation of the coagulation cascade in C1-inhibitor deficiencies. Blood 1997;89:3213–8.

[23] Cugno M, Hack CE, Boer JPD, et al. Generation of plasmin during acute attacks of hereditary angioedema. J Lab Clin Med 1993;121:38–43.

[24] Mast AE, Enghild JJ, Pizzo SV, et al. Analysis of the plasma elimination kinetics and conformational stabilities of native, proteinase-complexed, and reactive site cleaved serpins: comparison of alpha 1–proteinase inhibitor, alpha 1–antichymotrypsin, antithrombin III, alpha 2–antiplasmin, angiotensinogen, and ovalbumin. Biochemistry 1991;30: 1723–30.

[25] Bruch M, Weiss V, Engel J. Plasma serine proteinase inhibitors (serpins) exhibit major conformational changes and a large increase in conformational stability upon cleavage at their reactive sites. J Biol Chem 1988;263:16626–30.

[26] Batra PP, Sasa K, Ueki T, et al. Circular dichroic study of conformational changes in ovalbumin induced by modification of sulhydryl groups and disulfide reduction. J Protein Chem 1989;8:609–17.

[27] de Agostini A, Patston PA, Marottoli V, et al. A common neoepitope is created when the reactive center of C1-inhibitor is cleaved by plasma kallikrein, activated factor XII fragment, C1 esterase, or neutrophil elastase. J Clin Invest 1988;82:700–5.

[28] Nuijens JH, Huijbregts CCM, Eerenberg-Belmer AJM, et al. Quantification of plasma factor XIIa–C1-inhibitor and kallikrein–C1-inhibitor complexes in sepsis. Blood 1988;72: 1841–8.

[29] Nuijens JH, Eerenberg-Belmer AJM, Huijbregts CCM, et al. Proteolytic inactivation of plasma C1 inhibitor in sepsis. J Clin Invest 1989;84:443–50.

[30] Huntington JA, Read RJ, Carrell RW. Structure of a serpin-protease complex shows inhibition by deformation. Nature 2000;407:923–6.

[31] Patston PA, Gettins P, Beechem J, et al. Mechanism of serpin action: evidence that C1 inhibitor functions as a suicide substrate. Biochemistry 1991;30:8876–82.

[32] Bos IGA, Hack CE, Abrahams JP. Structural and functional aspects of C1-inhibitor. Immunobiology 2002;205:518–33.

[33] Bock SC, Skriver K, Nielsen E, et al. Human C1 inhibitor: primary structure, cDNA cloning, and chromosomal localization. Biochemistry 1986;25:4292–301.

[34] Coutinho M, Aulak KS, Davis AE III. Functional analysis of the serpin domain of C1 inhibitor. J Immunol 1994;153:3648–54.

[35] Liu D, Gu X, Scafidi J, Davis AE III. N-linked glycosylation is required for C1 inhibitor–mediated protection from endotoxin shock in mice. Infect Immun 2004;72(4): 1946–55.

[36] Liu D, Cramer CC, Scafidi J, Davis AE III. N-linked glycosylation at Asn3 and the positively charged residues within the amino terminal domain of C1 inhibitor are required for its interaction with Salmonella typhimurium lipopolysaccharide and lipid A. Infect Immun 2005;73:4478–87.

[37] Matsushita M, Endo Y, Fujita T. Cutting edge: complement-activating complex of ficolin and mannose-binding lectin-associated serine protease. J Immunol 2000;164:2281–4.

[38] Matsushita M, Thiel S, Jensenius JC, et al. Proteolytic activities of two types of mannose-binding lectin associated serine protease. J Immunol 2000;165:2637–42.

[39] Matsushita M, Endo Y, Hamasaki N, et al. Activation of the lectin complement pathway by ficolins. Int Immunopharmacol 2001;1:359–63.

[40] Ambrus G, Gal P, Kojima M, et al. Natural substrates and inhibitors of mannan-binding lectin-associated serine protease-1 and -2: a study on recombinant catalytic fragments. J Immunol 2003;170:1374-82.

[41] Jiang H, Wagner E, Zhang H, et al. Complement 1 inhibitor is a regulator of the alternative complement pathway. J Exp Med 2001;194:1609-16.

[42] Colman RW, Schmaier AH. Contact system: a vascular biology modulator with anticoagulant, profibrinolytic, antiadhesive, and proinflammatory attributes. Blood 1997;90:3819-43.

[43] Cochrane CG, Revak SD, Wuepper KD. Activation of Hageman factor in solid and fluid phases: a critical role of kallikrein. J Exp Med 1973;138:1564-83.

[44] Griffin JH. The role of surface in the surface-dependent activation of Hageman factor (blood coagulation factor XII). Proc Natl Acad Sci U S A 1978;75:1998-2002.

[45] Kaplan AP, Joseph K, Shibayama Y, et al. The intrinsic coagulation/kinin-forming cascade: assembly in plasma and cell surfaces in inflammation. Adv Immunol 1997;66:225-72.

[46] Kirby E, McDevitt PJ. The binding of bovine factor XII to kaolin. Blood 1983;61:652-9.

[47] Revak SD, Cochrane CG, Griffin JH. The binding and cleavage characteristics of human Hageman factor during contact activation: a comparison of normal plasma with plasma deficient in factor XI, prekallikrein or high molecular weight kininogen. J Clin Invest 1977;59: 1167-75.

[48] Mahdi F, Shariat-Madar Z, Todd RF III, et al. Expression and co-localization of cytokeratin 1 and urokinase plasminogen activator receptor on endothelial cells. Blood 2001;97: 2342-50.

[49] Joseph K, Ghebrehiwet B, Peerschke EIB, et al. Identification of the zinc-dependent endothelial cell binding protein for high molecular weight kininogen and factor XII: identity with the receptor that binds to the globular "heads" of C1q (gC1q-R). Proc Natl Acad Sci U S A 1996;93:8552-7.

[50] Joseph K, Kaplan AP. Formation of bradykinin: a major contributor to the innate inflammatory response. Adv Immunol 2005;86:159-208.

[51] Herwald H, Dedio J, Kellner R, et al. Isolation and characterization of the kininogen-binding protein p33 from endothelial cells. J Biol Chem 1996;271:13040-7.

[52] Colman RW, Pixley RA, Najamunnisa S, et al. Binding of high molecular weight kininogen to human endothelial cells is mediated via a site within domains 2 and 3 of the urokinase receptor. J Clin Invest 1997;100:1481-7.

[53] Hasan AAK, Zisman T, Schmaier AH. Identification of cytokeratin 1 as a binding protein and presentation receptor for kininogens on endothelial cells. Proc Natl Acad Sci U S A 1998;95:3615-20.

[54] Joseph K, Tholanikunnel BG, Kaplan AP. Activation of the bradykinin-forming cascade on endothelial cells: a role for heat shock protein 90. Int Immunopharmacol 2002;2:1851-9.

[55] Joseph K, Tholanikunnel BG, Kaplan AP. Heat shock protein 90 catalyzes activation of the prekallikrein-kininogen complex in the absence of factor XII. Proc Natl Acad Sci U S A 2002;99:896-900.

[56] Shariat-Madar Z, Mahdi F, Schmaier AH. Identification and characterization of prolylcarboxypeptidase as an endothelial cell prekallikrein activator. J Biol Chem 2002;277:17962-9.

[57] Shariat-Madar Z, Mahdi F, Schmaier AH. Assembly and activation of the plasma kallikrein/kinin system: a new interpretation. Int Immunopharmacol 2002;2:1841-9.

[58] Schmaier AH. The plasma kallikrein-kinin system counterbalances the renin-angiotensin system. J Clin Invest 2002;109:1007-9.

[59] Schmaier AH. The physiologic basis of assembly and activation of the plasma kallikrein/kinin system. Thromb Haemost 2004;91:1-3.

[60] Kramer J, Rosen F, Colten H, et al. Transinhibition of C1 inhibitor synthesis in type I hereditary angioneurotic edema. J Clin Invest 1993;91:1258-62.

[61] Ernst SC, Circolo A, Davis AE III, et al. Impaired production of both normal and mutant C1 inhibitor proteins in type I hereditary angioedema with a duplication in exon 8. J Immunol 1996;157:405-10.

[62] Brickman CM, Frank MM, Kaliner M. Urine-histamine levels in patients with hereditary angioedema (HAE). J Allergy Clin Immunol 1988;82:402–6.

[63] Colman RW. Activation of plasminogen by human plasma kallikrein. Biochem Biophys Res Commun 1969;35:273–9.

[64] Goldsmith GH, Saito H, Ratnoff OD. The activation of plasminogen by Hageman factor (factor XII) and Hageman factor fragments. J Clin Invest 1978;62:54–60.

[65] Revak SD, Cochrane CG, Bouma BN, et al. Surface and fluid-phase activities of two forms of activated Hageman factor produced during contact activation of plasma. J Exp Med 1978;147:719–29.

[66] Kaplan AP, Austen KF. A pre-albumin activator of prekallikrein. J Immunol 1970;105: 802–11.

[67] Ghebrehiwet B, Silverberg M, Kaplan AP. Activation of the classical pathway of complement by Hageman factor fragment. J Exp Med 1981;153:655–76.

[68] Donaldson DD. Mechanisms of activation of C1 esterase in hereditary angioneurotic edema plasma in vitro. The role of Hageman factor, a clot-promoting agent. J Exp Med 1968;127:411–29.

[69] Heinz HP, Loos M. Activation of the first component of complement, C1: comparison of the effect of sixteen different enzymes on C1. Immunobiology 1983;165:175–85.

[70] Francis CW, Brenner B, Leddy JP, et al. Angioedema during therapy with recombinant tissue plasminogen activator. Br J Haematol 1991;77:562–3.

[71] Hoffmeister HM, Szabo S, Kastner C, et al. Thrombolytic therapy in acute myocardial infarction: comparison of procoagulant effects of streptokinase and alteplase regimens with focus on the kallikrein system and plasmin. Circulation 1998;98:2527–33.

[72] Molinaro G, Gervais N, Adam A. Biochemical basis of angioedema associated with recombinant tissue plasminogen activator treatment: an in vitro experimental approach. Stroke 2002;33:1712–6.

[73] Donaldson VH, Rosen FS. Action of complement in hereditary angioneurotic edema: the role of C'1 esterase. J Clin Invest 1964;43:2204–13.

[74] Carpenter CB, Ruddy S, Shehadeh IH, et al. Complement metabolism in man: hypercatabolism of the fourth (C4) and third (C3) components in patients with renal allograft rejection and hereditary angioedema (HAE). J Clin Invest 1969;48:1495–505.

[75] Austen KF, Sheffer AL. Detection of hereditary angioneurotic edema by demonstration of a profound reduction in the second component of human complement. N Engl J Med 1965; 272:649–56.

[76] Quastel M, Harrison R, Cicardi M, et al. Behavior in vivo of normal and dysfunctional C1 inhibitor in normal subjects and patients with hereditary angioneurotic edema. J Clin Invest 1983;71:1041–6.

[77] Lachmann P, Rosen F. The catabolism of C1-inhibitor and the pathogenesis of hereditary angioedema. Acta Pathol Microbiol Immunol Scand 1984;284:35–9.

[78] Laurell AB, Lindgren J, Malmros I, et al. Enzymatic and immunochemical estimation of C1 esterase inhibitor in sera from patients with hereditary angioedema. Scand J Clin Lab Invest 1969;24:221–5.

[79] Laurell AB, Martensson U, Sjoholm AG. C1 subcomponent complexes in normal and pathological sera studied by crossed immunoelectrophoresis. Acta Pathol Microbiol Scand 1976;84:455–64.

[80] Donaldson VH, Ratnoff OD, Silva WDD, et al. Permeability-increasing activity in hereditary angioneurotic edema plasma. J Clin Invest 1969;48:642–53.

[81] Donaldson VH, Merler E, Rosen FS, et al. A polypeptide kinin in hereditary angioneurotic edema plasma: role of complement in its formation. J Lab Clin Med 1970;76:986.

[82] Donaldson VH. Kinin formation in hereditary angioneurotic edema (HANE) plasma. Int Arch Allergy Appl Immunol 1973;45:206–9.

[83] Davies GE, Lowe JS. A permeability factor released from guinea pig serum by antigen-antibody precipitates. Brit J Exp Pathol 1960;41:335–44.

[84] Klemperer MR, Donaldson VH, Rosen FS. Effect of C1 esterase on vascular permeability in man: studies in normal and complement-deficient individuals and in patients with hereditary angioneurotic edema. J Clin Invest 1968;47:604–11.

[85] Ratnoff OD, Lepow IH. Complement as a mediator of inflammation. Enhancement of vascular permeability by purified C'1 esterase. J Exp Med 1963;118:681–98.

[86] Davis AE III, Davis JS IV, Rabson AR, et al. Homozygous C3 deficiency: detection of C3 by radioimmunoassay. Clin Immunol Immunopathol 1977;8:543–50.

[87] Strang CJ, Auerbach KS, Rosen FS. C1s-induced vascular permeability in C2-deficient guinea pigs. J Immunol 1986;137:631–5.

[88] Strang C, Cholin S, Spragg J, et al. Angioedema induced by a peptide derived from complement component C2. J Exp Med 1988;168:1685–98.

[89] Donaldson V, Rosen F, Bing D. Role of the second component of complement (C2) and plasmin in kinin release in hereditary angioneurotic edema (H.A.N.E.). Trans Assoc Am Physicians 1977;90:174–83.

[90] Smith M, Kerr M. Cleavage of the second component of complement by plasma proteases: implications in hereditary C1-inhibitor deficiency. Immunology 1985;56:561–70.

[91] Curd JG, Prograis LJ Jr, Cochrane CG. Detection of active kallikrein in induced blister fluids of hereditary angioedema patients. J Exp Med 1980;152:742–7.

[92] Schapira M, Silver LD, Scott CF, et al. Prekallikrein activation and high-molecular-weight kininogen consumption in hereditary angioedema. N Engl J Med 1983;308:1050–3.

[93] Curd JG, Yelvington M, Burridge N, et al. Generation of bradykinin during incubation of hereditary angioedema plasma [abstract]. Mol Immunol 1982;19:1365.

[94] Fields T, Ghebrewihet B, Kaplan A. Kinin formation in hereditary angioedema plasma: evidence against kinin derivation from C2 and in support of spontaneous formation of bradykinin. J Allergy Clin Immunol 1983;72:54–60.

[95] Berrettini M, Lammle B, White T, et al. Detection of in vitro and in vivo cleavage of high molecular weight kininogen in human plasma by immunoblotting with monoclonal antibodies. Blood 1986;68:455–62.

[96] Lammle B, Zuraw BL, Heeb MJ, et al. Detection and quantitation of cleaved and uncleaved high molecular weight kininogen in plasma by ligand blotting with radiolabeled plasma prekallikrein or factor XI. Thromb Haemost 1988;59:151–61.

[97] Nielsen EW, Johansen HT, Hogasen K, et al. Activation of the complement, coagulation, fibrinolytic and kallikrein-kinin systems during attacks of hereditary angioedema. Scand J Immunol 1996;44:185–92.

[98] Cugno M, Cicardi M, Coppola R, et al. Activation of factor XII and cleavage of high molecular weight kininogen during acute attacks in hereditary and acquired C1-inhibitor deficiencies. Immunopharmacology 1996;33:361–4.

[99] Buhler R, Hovinga JK, Aebi-Huber I, et al. Improved detection of proteolytically cleaved high molecular weight kininogen by immunoblotting using an antiserum against its reduced 47 kDa light chain. Blood Coagul Fibrinolysis 1995;6:223–32.

[100] Shoemaker LR, Schurman SJ, Donaldson VH, et al. Hereditary angioneurotic edema: characterization of plasma kinin and vascular permeability–enhancing activities. Clin Exp Immunol 1994;95:22–8.

[101] Nussberger J, Cugno M, Amstutz C, et al. Plasma bradykinin in angio-oedema. Lancet 1998;351:1693–7.

[102] Wisnieski JJ, Knauss TC, Yike I, et al. Unique C1 inhibitor dysfunction in a kindred without angioedema. I. A mutant C1 inhibitor that inhibits C1s but not C1r. J Immunol 1994;152:3199–209.

[103] Zahedi R, Bissler JJ, Davis AE III, et al. Unique C1 inhibitor dysfunction in a kindred without angioedema. II. Identification of an Ala443-Val substitution and functional analysis of the recombinant mutant protein. J Clin Invest 1995;95:1299–305.

[104] Zahedi R, Wisnieski J, Davis AE III. Role of the P2 residue of complement 1 inhibitor (Ala443) in determination of target protease specificity. J Immunol 1997;159:983–8.

[105] Zahedi R, MacFarlane RC, Wisnieski JJ, Davis AE III. C1 inhibitor: analysis of the role of amino acid residues within the reactive center loop in target protease recognition. J Immunol 2001;167:1500–6.

[106] Han ED, MacFarlane RC, Mulligan AN, et al. Increased vascular permeability in C1 inhibitor–deficient mice is mediated by the bradykinin type 2 receptor. J Clin Invest 2002;109: 1057–63.

[107] Agostini AD, Lijnen HR, Pixley RA, et al. Inactivation of factor XII active fragment in normal plasma. Predominant role of C1-inhibitor. J Clin Invest 1984;73:1542–9.

[108] Dyax Corporation; 2004. Available at: www.dyax.com. Accessed July 6, 2006.

[109] Jerini. Available at: www.jerini.com. Accessed July 6, 2006.

ELSEVIER
SAUNDERS

Immunol Allergy Clin N Am
26 (2006) 653–668

IMMUNOLOGY
AND ALLERGY
CLINICS
OF NORTH AMERICA

Hereditary Angioedema: The Clinical Syndrome and its Management in the United States

Michael M. Frank, MD

Duke University Medical Center, Box 2611, Durham, NC 27710, USA

Hereditary angioedema (HAE) is an episodic swelling disease with autosomal Mendelian dominant inheritance. One of the oldest descriptions of the disease is from the 1840s by Graves, who clearly described patients with episodic angioedema [1]. In 1882, Quincke described a constellation of angioedema symptoms including peripheral swelling and self-limited attacks of abdominal pain; the disease is known in Europe as Quincke's disease [2]. His original description includes concern about compromise of the airway. Because the attacks he described usually lasted a matter of hours rather than days, the length of time we commonly associate with HAE today, we cannot be completely certain that the attacks described 124 years ago were hereditary angioedema. A few years later in 1888, Osler described the disease observed in each of five generations of a family and identified the autosomal dominant inheritance that we now associate with the disease [3].

Hereditary angioedema is characterized by sporadic episodic swelling, usually of the hands and feet, but occasionally of the genitalia, face, tongue, and larynx [4]. The swelling is due to edema of the dermal layers of the skin caused by leakage of plasma from capillary or more likely postcapillary venules and is often not well circumscribed. It is described as brawny, nonpitting edema. The swelling is never associated with pain, although the swelling alone with loss of flexibility of the tissues may cause some discomfort, if it involves the tissues around a joint. Patients commonly also have episodic swelling of the wall of the bowel leading to severe abdominal pain. The abdominal pain is often spasmodic rather than steady and presumably increases with each peristaltic wave; this suggests that there is an element of bowel obstruction associated with the attacks. In many patients, vomiting, particularly early in the attack, is a regular feature of the episode. Patients

---

E-mail address: frank007@mc.duke.edu

0889-8561/06/$ - see front matter © 2006 Elsevier Inc. All rights reserved.
doi:10.1016/j.iac.2006.09.005
immunology.theclinics.com

may have constipation associated with an attack, but this is not constant and diarrhea is sometimes observed. On physical exam the abdomen often has few bowel sounds at the height of an abdominal attack, but this is also not constant, and rushing bowel sounds may be heard. Although the patient usually has a protuberant abdomen with a great deal of tenderness and at times rebound tenderness and guarding, this is not a rigid surgical abdominal exam.

Many males describe episodic swelling in the genital area with swelling involving the testes and penis. In my experience the frequency of genital attacks is low, but a high proportion of males have had at least some genital attacks. In general, swelling, although at times uncomfortable, is not life threatening, except when it involves the airway. However, when the swelling does involve the airway it can lead to asphyxiation and death. In studies outlining the clinical syndrome, which we reported in 1976, we noted that about one third of untreated patients, identified by our patients as family members with the disease, had a history of asphyxiation [4]. Clearly this is a high figure, because the family members who would be remembered are the ones who had the most severe disease, but nevertheless, this is a sobering number. Attacks of abdominal angioedema, although not life threatening, cause severe pain and patients are often taken to the emergency room and operated on because of the severity of the clinical symptoms.

In the average patient, attacks grow more severe for about a day and a half and then clear over another day and a half, but there are many exceptions to this rule. There are patients whose attacks generally last less than 24 hours, and there are patients whose abdominal pain attacks last 4 or 5 days and whose peripheral swelling attacks last on average as many as 9 days. Thus, the variability of this disease is really quite remarkable.

Angioedema attacks are often heralded by a prodrome. At times the prodrome consists of a feeling of tingling in the area where the attack will start for an hour or so before the attack. Presumably this represents the release of mediators that will induce capillary or postcapillary venule leakage, ultimately leading to attacks. Nevertheless, there are rare patients who have no prodrome and some patients who have prodromes for as long as 24 hours before the onset of an attack. At the start of an attack, some patients will have erythema marginatum, which they often describe as red circles on the skin. This rash, which often occurs at the start of an attack, is nonpruritic and not raised, and patients often remark that they would not know they had the rash unless they saw it or someone pointed it out. Again, they are not an invariant feature of the disease; about one third of patients have erythema marginatum at the time of an attack.

Although attacks are sporadic and often do not have a clear initiating cause, many patients note that pressure will often bring on an attack. Thus, a person who mows the lawn with a power lawn mower may find that the hands swell up or a woman who is a seamstress and uses a pair of scissors for a long time may note that the hand with which she used the scissors swells up. In general, attacks are not symmetrical and often extend locally, but they may pass from one hand to a foot or one hand to the other hand, and so forth. A second precipitating cause that patients notice is emotional stress. Often they find that for unknown reasons at times of tension or high stress, their attack frequency increases. Thus, a student who has a great deal of stress surrounding an examination may have an attack before the examination. A woman confided in me that in an unhappy marriage, she had many attacks and when she got divorced and remarried to a man with whom she was more compatible, her attack frequency decreased markedly. In our initial series we noted that about one third of patients noted stress-precipitating attacks and one third noted trauma as a cause.

Attacks usually begin in childhood, but they may begin at any age. There are patients with HAE whose first attacks began at age 90. Presumably they had the biochemical abnormality all of their lives and something brought on the sudden conversion to attacks of HAE at this late age. Often initiation of use of angiotensin-converting enzyme (ACE) inhibitors is the event that activates long-standing quiescent disease [5]. ACE is important in the catabolism of bradykinin and presumably by inhibiting this enzyme, the inhibitor precipitates the bradykinin-induced attacks. In general, however, attacks start in childhood and are quite mild. Because children often have attacks of abdominal pain associated with gastrointestinal viruses and so forth, they are often not remarked upon by the patient's family or pediatrician. However, at the time of puberty, it is common for attacks to become much more severe and it is then that the full-blown syndrome develops. Presumably, the attacks are of equal severity and frequency in men and women as predicted by the autosomal dominant inheritance, but I and most physicians who have taken care of many patients over the years have noted a preponderance of women coming for care. This may represent selection bias but may be a reflection of hormonal influences on disease severity. Early on, we noted that estrogens cause attack frequency to increase and for attacks to become more severe [4,6]. These estrogens may be of many types including artificial estrogens and natural products like Premarin. Some women are exquisitely sensitive to estrogens, and very tiny amounts of estrogen taken to relieve symptoms of menopause may be enough to increase attack frequency and severity; it is occasionally true that a woman can be treated by simply taking her off estrogen-containing birth control pills. Many women note that attack frequencies are highest at the time of menstruation.

The most debilitating attacks experienced by patients are the abdominal pain attacks discussed earlier. These attacks of edema are never associated with bowel wall necrosis, but may be sufficiently severe to cause obstruction of the gastrointestinal (GI) tract. On GI series during attack, there is usually spiculation or thumb printing of the mucosa, representing edema of the ruggai of the GI tract. Occasionally, repeated attacks preventing adequate biliary drainage can lead to gallbladder disease, or attacks preventing pancreatic drainage can lead to pancreatitis.

The most dangerous attacks are those that affect the airways. Often these attacks start in the mouth and extend to the larynx. Since trauma can sometimes bring on an attack, these patients learn to fear the dentist because they may have particular difficulty following injection of Novocain into the gums. Their teeth may be in poor repair. The attacks are presumed to be the same as those that affect peripheral sites, but because the airway, particularly in the region of the vocal cords, is constricted, a relatively small amount of edema may do great damage. As with peripheral attacks, these attacks usually increase in severity for about 1 and a half days and then resolve over the same period of time but again this may be variable.

HAE is often grouped with the allergic disorders, but there is no evidence that it is allergic in nature. A few of the patients have urticaria at times, but it is by no means common and one must assume that the incidence of allergies, hives, and so forth, in the HAE population is the same as in the general population. Patients can go for extended periods of time without HAE attacks and then once again become far more severe, and it is not known why the disease tends to wax and wane. Although this has not been carefully studied, one gets the impression that in certain families the pattern of attacks may be similar. For example, in my experience there are families that have mostly abdominal pain attacks and even an occasional family with an unusually high incidence of HAE affecting the throat. Patients with only abdominal attacks have been reported [7]. An interesting point that has not been studied in detail is that patients noted, before any useful therapy was available, that after a severe attack they often were attack free for a period of time. Thus, if they needed dental work done, they might wait until they had a very severe attack and then over the next several days go to the dentist, when they would find that they would be resistant to attacks and they could safely undergo extractions and other procedures. The reasons for this are unknown.

Patients with HAE in general do well with pregnancy. Usually their attack frequency is unchanged in the first trimester, but by the time the second trimester starts, their attack frequency is decreasing and they note that their third trimester is the best period that they have had in years. I have never seen a patient have an attack of HAE associated with the trauma of delivery, but it is not uncommon to have patients develop HAE attacks 3 to 7 days after the delivery is completed. Although we speak here of average patients, I have seen patients get worse during pregnancy more than once and when this happens, it represents a difficult management problem. In a few patients attacks have become so severe during the last trimester of pregnancy that we treated them with infusions of fresh frozen plasma three times per week to keep them relatively free of symptoms (see section on prophylaxis). I have no information that would explain why in a very few patients attacks become much more severe in late pregnancy, but I have wondered whether these patients might have an area of necrotic placenta that activates an inflammatory reaction, further catabolism of C1 Inhibitor, and an increase in attacks.

Although this has never been carefully evaluated, some investigators believe that attacks become less severe as patients age.

A question arises as to whether patients with HAE are not healthy psychologically. Clearly many patients are healthy psychologically, but many people have been struck by the fact that a subgroup of patients appears to have more psychological problems than might be expected. Patients at times have seen family members die of asphyxiation because of a disease that they themselves have, and other patients know of family members who have died. This I am sure leads to psychological difficulties. In any case, some years ago with Mary Huber, RN, we had formal psychological testing performed on a group of patients. They proved to demonstrate more impulsive behavior than a healthy patient group. Several patients have told me that they don't feel healthy psychologically at the start of an attack and I cannot but wonder whether the mediators that are responsible for attacks affect the brain.

Pathophysiology of hereditary angioedema

This topic will not be covered in detail here; see the article by Davis in this issue. In 1962 Landerman and colleagues [8] studied patients with hereditary angioedema, using what would now be considered crude technology, and suggested that kinin generation in their blood might be poorly regulated, and that the patients had an inherited defect in an inhibitor to a permeability factor, probably kallikrein. In retrospect this was an important observation. However, the great breakthrough in our understanding of angioedema came with the important work of Dr. Virginia Donaldson in 1962 [9] Dr. Donaldson was conducting research in laboratories at Case Western Reserve Medical Center, close to those of Dr. Irwin Lepow. Dr. Lepow was investigating the properties of a newly defined protein that controlled the activation and activity of the complement protein C1. C1 is a complement system protein that circulates as an inactive precursor and is activated during certain immunologic reactions. At that time the new protein was termed C1 esterase inhibitor, because the assay in use for C1, the enzyme that was inhibited by the new protein, was cleavage of a synthetic ester substrate. Currently, the name has been shortened to C1 inhibitor. Lepow had prepared antibody to C1 inhibitor and Dr. Donaldson studied a variety of patients including patients with HAE for the level of protein in their blood. She made the seminal observation that patients with HAE have low circulating levels of C1 inhibitor, an observation that has stood the test of time [9]. This finding allowed for studies of the pathophysiology of HAE that have continued to this time (see chapter on pathophysiology). Further studies of Rosen and colleagues [10], evaluating a group of patients with HAE, demonstrated that 85% of patients (Type 1) have low levels of C1 inhibitor and 15% of patients (type 2) have normal or elevated levels of a poorly functioning protein. Presumably type 1 patients have a gene that leads to no C1

INH synthesis or failure to secrete protein and type 2 defects lead to a secreted but nonfunctioning protein.

The action of C1 inhibitor on C1 is twofold. It controls the rate of activation of C1 and it inactivates the active protein. C1 is the first protein component of the classical complement cascade. It circulates as an enzymatically inactive three-part molecule, C1q, C1r, and C1s, the parts held together in the presence of Ca^{++}. C1 binds via the C1q subunit to antigen-antibody complexes of the correct sort and becomes activated, that is it develops enzymatic activity. The function of activated C1 is to cleave the next two proteins in the classical complement pathway sequence, C4 and C2. It was quickly noted that patients with HAE almost always have low levels of C4 and C2, even between attacks. A rare patient has normal C4 and C2 levels between attacks. The protein that follows C2 in the sequence of steps in the complement cascade is C3 and the level of C3 is virtually always normal in these patients [4,11]. This reflects the fact that there are both circulating and cell membrane–bound proteins that regulate the level of C3 and turn off untoward activation of enzymes that would cleave C3 and lower its level in serum. Thus, in general, patients with HAE have normal C1 levels, low levels of C4 and C2, and normal levels of C3. Their level of C1 inhibitor is usually in the range of about one-third the lower limit of normal, but again, there is considerable variability in this level from patient to patient.

With the understanding that patients with HAE have constant activation of C4 and C2, attention turned to these two proteins as the possible source of the mediators causing this disease. It seemed extremely likely that a mediator was released in blood or tissue when this regulatory protein was at low levels or not properly functioning and the likeliest candidates for the source were C4 and C2. A series of papers were written that suggested that a cleavage product, C2b, could be acted upon by plasmin, another protein found to be inhibited by C1 INH, to create a peptide termed C2 kinin that mediated capillary leakage; C2 peptide became a candidate for the cause of attacks [12,13]. The question of histamine contributing to attacks was raised as well. Brickman and colleagues [14] reported that histamine concentration does not rise in the urine during attacks and appears to be normal at all times, confirming the suggestion that, unlike allergic diseases, this disease is not allergic in nature and not due to histamine release and mast cell degranulation.

Studies of the C1 inhibitor led to an understanding of the fact that this protein inhibits many of the mediator cascades in serum. These actions of C1 inhibitor are reviewed elsewhere in this issue.

There are a number of issues related to the pathophysiology of HAE that are not quite clear and may be important in the future as we sort out the various aspects of the basis of this disease: It was shown early on that the level of C1 inhibitor is not associated with the severity of disease, although all patients have low C1 inhibitor or a nonfunctioning protein [4]. In other words, patients who have a mildly decreased level may have very severe clinical symptoms and patients who have an extremely severe depression may have a very mild case of the disease. The reasons for this are unclear. Moreover, subcutaneous injection of bradykinin into experimental animals or humans leads to severe pain, because it stimulates pain fibers. Patients with HAE have no pain associated with attacks. Injection of bradykinin into animals causes hypotension. Patients with HAE rarely become hypotensive unless they have had a severe fluid shift from the intravascular space into edematous bowel or other tissues.

Another fascinating finding is that patients with HAE have a higher than normal incidence of autoimmune diseases, although the diseases are often mild [15–17]. The type of autoimmune disease is quite variable and appears to reflect the genotype and underlying predisposition of the patient. Disease can range from systemic lupus erythmatosus (SLE), to hypo or hyperthyroidism, to inflammatory bowel disease. Careful study of a large group of patients led to the finding that these patients have an elevated level of T helper cells and that the degree of elevation was inversely correlated with the plasma C4 level [18]. Complement activation is known to affect the afferent limb of the immune response and presumably constant activation of complement in this patient group leads to low C4, increased T helper cell activation, and an elevated incidence of autoimmunity.

Treatment of hereditary angioedema

For convenience, therapy of HAE is usually divided into chronic long-term therapy, short-term prophylactic therapy, and treatment of acute attacks.

Chronic long-term therapy

It is humbling to note that an approach to chronic treatment of HAE using methyltestosterone was detailed in the literature several years before any discussion of pathophysiology began and before the importance of C1 inhibitor was noted [19]. Because the reported therapy fit no reasonable theory as to why it should be effective, and because it was of a class of drug thought to be unlikely to be effective in angioedema, the observation was lost for over a decade. In 1960, Spaulding [19] described a single family with HAE treated with methyltestosterone. They reported a limited double-blind study suggesting that the drug was quite effective in this family; however, this method of therapy never came into use and even the report's existence was lost to investigators in the field. With the observation that estrogens made HAE more severe, the fact that patients with HAE improved during pregnancy and had no trouble with the trauma of delivery, and the increase in clinical symptoms at the time of puberty, my group first attempted a study of progesterone in the treatment of HAE. Although we never reported our findings, we found that patients all felt better on progesterone therapy, but in our small group of patients the attack frequency did not decrease. We then turned to the study of Danazol, an impeded androgen that was being developed for administration to women as a contraceptive [20]. This drug was a gonadotropin inhibitor and therefore could be expected to decrease estrogen levels in both males and females. Because it was an impeded androgen being developed as a female contraceptive, it had little androgenic activity and could be used in most women. It was for this reason that we chose to do a double-blind study of Danazol. At about the same time others were studying Stanazolol and methyltestosterone for the treatment of HAE. Our study design, developed by a brilliant statistician Dr. David Alling, was of particular interest. Patients all served as their own controls. Patients were given a 28-day course of drug or placebo. If, during the course, the patients had an attack they were considered a drug failure and went on to the next blind course. The patients were asked whether they were taking drug or placebo and the courses were sufficiently short that they could not identify the courses that included drug. The results were striking (Table 1). These were severely affected patients and almost every placebo course was attended by an attack. All but one course on drug was attack free. Thus we found that Danazol was highly effective in treatment. Similarly, all of the studies of impeded androgens confirmed the findings of Spalding [21–23]. Further work has suggested that the only androgens that are useful in therapy are methylated androgens that must be given orally. Testosterone, for example testosterone patches, do not prevent attacks of HAE. In our studies, we were surprised to find that not only was the drug, Danazol, extremely effective in treatment, but in most patients, it led to a marked increase in the blood levels of C1 inhibitor. This was associated with clinical and biochemical improvement. With the increased levels of C1 inhibitor, the C4 level tended to return to normal and the clinical symptoms disappeared. Thus, androgens appeared to be causing the synthesis of a protein known to be produced in the liver. We found the synthesis of all proteins produced in the liver is not increased; for example, the blood levels of albumin and C3 were not changed. Although some studies suggest that impeded androgens increase messenger RNA for C1 inhibitor in peripheral blood cells, this is not confirmed in other studies, and there is still no definitive study of the effect of impeded androgens on C1 inhibitor synthesis [24–26]. Nevertheless, most investigators assume that increased hepatic synthesis of C1 inhibitor is its mechanism of action. It became clear that it was impossible to predict in

Table 1
Treatment results

	Total courses	Attack-free courses	Attacks
Danazol	42	41	1
Placebo	46	3	43
Total	88	44	44

any individual patient the dose of androgen that would be required to reliably decrease or terminate attacks [27]. In the case of Danazol, there are rare individuals who do not respond to 800 mg a day and others who respond very satisfactorily to 50 mg once a week. We tend to start treatment at 200 mg three times a day, because this dose almost always prevents attacks and the patient is therefore reassured and relaxes. We then progressively lower the dosage slowly over months to determine the lowest dosage that will prevent attacks (Table 2). All impeded androgens have a number of potentially important side effects including masculinization, headaches, lack of libido or increased libido, hair gain or loss, liver function abnormalities including possible peliosis hepatic, and abnormalities in serum lipids (Table 3) [28–30]. Danazol can induce hematuria caused by low-level cystitis or bladder telangectasia [28]. These side effects have tended to be mild and in my hands the abnormalities have disappeared when the drug has been stopped. When faced with mild transaminase elevations or minimal hematuria, we have at times continued treatment, when the only other choice was resumption of attacks, and our patients have never gotten into trouble. In particular we have never had hematuria develop into hemorrhagic cystitis as sometimes occurs in patients on Cytoxan therapy. Obviously, the various untoward possibilities must be discussed with patients in detail. I have had no luck in switching patients from one androgen to another to avoid side effects.

Despite the side effects, most patients are so pleased to be offered a drug that is functionally active and relieves their symptoms that they insist on facing up to the dangers and taking the drug. Androgens are not useful in terminating ongoing attacks, since it often takes at least 48 hours for the androgen to begin to have an effect.

A variety of impeded androgens are now available in the United States. This author has most experience with Danazol. However, others have used other impeded androgens and there clearly are patients who prefer one impeded androgen over another. Oxandrolone has been recommended, especially in children [31]. We have tried to switch from one impeded androgen to another and have never been able to decrease drug toxicity by this method.

Table 2
Effective therapeutic dose of danazol[a]

Danazol dose	% with clinical response
600 mg	95
400 mg	88
300 mg	58
200 mg	11

[a] At the lowest effective therapeutic dose there may be no evidence of a biochemical response.

Table 3
Side effects of danazol therapy

Side effect	No.	%
Abnormal liver function tests	9	16
Hematuria	9	16
Myopathy	21	38
Myalgias, cramps	17	30
Elevated CPK	11	20
Headache	7	16
Abnormal menses requiring Rx	5	13
Decreased libido	5	9
Hair loss	7	13
Anxiety reactions	18	32

Abbreviation: CPK, creative phosphokinase

Following the observation of Spaulding, but before the other impeded androgens were found to be effective in the treatment of HAE, it was noted that epsilon aminocaproic acid (EACA) is effective in the treatment of the disease [32–34]. Because it was believed that plasmin acting on C2 might generate the angioedema causing peptides, it was decided to use this plasmin inhibitor. In an empiric noncontrolled study it was found that symptoms of angioedema were improved. This was confirmed in a limited number of patients, first in Sweden and then in England [33,34] (Table 4). We performed the first double-blind study that confirmed the activity of epsilon aminocaproic acid in the treatment of this disease [35]. Similar to the Danazol study, patients were treated with drug or placebo for 1-month courses and each patient served as his or her own control. There were two attacks in 21 courses of EACA and each of 24 courses on placebo ended in an attack. There was no change in C1 inhibitor or C4 titer during drug treatment. Thus, the drug proved to be very effective. A dose-finding study suggested that most patients respond to about 8 g EACA per day. Others showed that tranexamic acid, a circularized relative of EACA, is far more effective on a per milligram basis [36]. It was interesting that in our studies, patients on EACA noted the prodrome of HAE attack, but the attack spread slowly. This

Table 4
Treatment of hereditary angioedema with epsilon amincaproic acid

Case (Sex)	Age, y	Courses with EACA		Courses with placebo	
		Without attacks	With attacks	Without attacks	With attacks
1 (M)	22	2	2	0	4
2 (F)	30	5	0	0	5
3 (F)	47	5	0	0	5
4 (M)	57	4	0	0	5
5 (F)	22	3	0	0	5

Data from Frank MM, Sergent JS, Kane MA, et al. Epsilon aminocaproic acid therapy of hereditary angioneurotic edema: a double-blind study. N Engl J Med 1972;286(15):808–12.

was quite different from the situation with the impeded androgens, where the patient noted no prodrome and no attack. In our hands, EACA has proven to be a very difficult drug to use. We found early on that patients sometimes develop severe muscle toxicity on EACA. One of our early patients had to be carried to the phone because she had severe weakness from EACA, although she was having relief from her HAE. Work-up showed a markedly elevated CPK (creatine phosphokinase) and aldolase. The weakness and biochemical abnormalities cleared when the EACA was discontinued. The reason for the severe muscle toxicity noted with these drugs is unknown. It is interesting that even on androgens, some patients will detect muscle toxicity and I think it quite likely that patients with HAE have a muscle problem as well as an angioedema problem, although its nature has never been clearly defined. As with impeded androgens, there is a considerable time lag (probably 48 hours) before the effect of EACA in controlling angioedema is manifest. Since over 90% of the drug is excreted in the urine in 6 hours the reasons for this are unclear. Since the drug treatment does not lead to an increase in the level of C4, I do not believe that the mechanism of action of this agent is to act as a C1 inhibitor.

Chronic disease treatment for HAE is satisfactory for most patients, but it requires daily treatment. However, both androgens and plasmin inhibitors are not useful in some patients. The treatments available are not proven to be safe in pregnant women where masculinization of the fetus on androgens can occur. In some women the side effects are intolerable. Finally some patients do not respond to therapy.

The article in this issue by Davis discusses C1 inhibitor, the characteristics of the protein, and its mechanism of action and this material will not be reviewed here. The C1 inhibitor gene has eight exons, four of them preceded by ALU sequences. It is believed that one reason for large deletions in the gene is improper alignment of the gene on chromosomes during meiosis. This would lead to a truncated protein ultimately leading to no product. A large number of mutations over much of the C1 inhibitor molecule have been described in patients. It has been found that those patients with type 2 HAE for the most part have single point mutations near the active site, thus preventing the formation of a C1 inhibitor enzyme complex. Treatment of acute attacks with C1 inhibitor is discussed below, but there is at least one report that suggests that weekly C1 inhibitor infusions are effective as chronic prophylactic therapy [37].

Short-term prophylaxis to prevent attacks

There are times when patients with HAE require short-term prophylaxis to prevent attacks. For example, if a patient is to undergo dental surgery, it is essential that attacks be prevented. Similarly, if a patient is in an automobile accident and is not having an attack, it may be prudent to prevent attacks from occurring. In these situations in which prophylaxis is important, fresh frozen plasma has been used successfully to prevent attacks [38–40]. Two units of fresh frozen plasma given the night before surgery or even in many cases on the day of surgery have prevented attacks, and it has been possible to treat patients as if they did not have HAE.

Presumably, the fresh frozen plasma replaces the missing C1 inhibitor, which acts to control attacks. As discussed in section on therapy of acute attacks, substrates that can be acted on to release mediators such as high-molecular-weight kininogen may be present in the infused plasma and may exacerbate an ongoing attack, but if the patient has no signs of an attack at the time of the infusion, this is not a problem. In our published studies we infused the plasma the night before surgery to be certain that the molecule had sufficient time to leave the circulation and enter the extracellular space, but recent experience suggests that this is not necessary. Since the half-life of C1 inhibitor in the circulation of patients is about 40 to 60 hours, it is not reasonable to expect the effectiveness to last more than about 3 days, although experience suggests that the effect of the protein may actually last longer.

There are reports in the literature of using androgen or plasmin inhibitors as prophylaxis in these situations [41,42]. Androgen as noted in the section on chronic therapy is useful as chronic therapy in preventing attacks of HAE and is not useful for acute attacks. We have elected not to use attenuated androgens for the most part in prophylaxis of attacks. An occasional patient will have an attack on adequate chronic prophylactic therapy. For example, I have seen a patient develop complete respiratory obstruction on chronic Danazol, 600 mg per day. I therefore am uneasy about using chronic androgen therapy to prevent attacks in potentially life-threatening situations, when there is no adequate back-up therapy. Nevertheless, there are those who have used it successfully. In a similar vein, I do not use plasmin inhibitors as prophylaxis for procedures, although others have reported success with this treatment. There is no question that patients can have attacks on plasmin inhibitor therapy and again at this time there is no adequate therapy. Once C1 inhibitor or other agents that reliably terminate attacks is available, it may be reasonable to use attenuated androgens or plasmin inhibitors with the understanding that if an attack starts, the patient will be treated rapidly with one of these other agents.

Therapy of acute attacks

In the United States, therapy of acute attacks is the area that has received the least attention and is most unsatisfactory. In the United States, patients receive supportive therapy. They are treated with epinephrine, which in this investigator's opinion often has a mild, but not dependable, effect in limiting attacks, being beneficial particularly early in attacks. Patients are also given antihistamines for sedation and are usually given glucocorticoids, although there is no evidence that glucocorticoids have efficacy. I treat patients with

EACA as well (16 g a day for the first day, falling back to 8 g a day), not because the EACA terminates attacks but because the physician can be assured that 48 hours later the attack will begin to resolve. Since EACA is available in intravenous form in most hospital pharmacies and has very little toxicity in this acute setting, there is little reason for not adding it to therapy, unless there is a contraindication. Contraindications would include advanced age, previous thrombosis, or procoagulant state. Clearly, airway management is the most important aspect of treatment of acute attacks of HAE and patients are given nasotracheal intubation if possible, before there is complete airway obstruction, or a tracheotomy. Inability to swallow secretions, or a change in the tone of the voice, often are indicators of impending airway obstruction. Acute attacks of abdominal pain are usually treated with narcotics. The latter are the only agents that relieve the acute pain. Patients with HAE are particularly prone to develop narcotic addiction, and care must be taken to prevent the overuse of narcotics in this patient group. We particularly try to avoid the use of Demerol, a favorite of the addicted patients. As mentioned, epinephrine sometimes has an effect and we use it for abdominal as well as peripheral attacks. Narcotics given very early in an attack for unknown reasons may terminate the attack.

In 1969 Pickering and his colleagues [43] published a report of treatment of acute angioedema attacks with fresh frozen plasma and many patients will recount successful treatment of attacks with fresh frozen plasma. Those of us who have taken care of many patients with HAE in acute, sometimes life-threatening situations have noted that a few patients get worse following fresh frozen plasma. Presumably, as discussed above, substrate for the various active enzymes is present in fresh frozen plasma and the replacement of fresh frozen plasma replaces substrate as well as the inhibitor. Depending on ratio of substrate and inhibitor, the edema formation may get worse before it gets better. Since in this country we do not have a satisfactory treatment for acute attacks of HAE, many of those who have taken care of many patients feel that it is undesirable to treat a patient with fresh frozen plasma at the time of a possible acute life-threatening attack.

When it became apparent that patients with HAE have low levels of C1 inhibitor, the idea of using C1 inhibitor to terminate attacks was advanced. In the United States, our group working with the American Red Cross developed a C1 inhibitor preparation, which we studied in a group of patients with HAE [44]. We reported in 1980 that the preparation successfully terminated attacks in a non–double-blind study. Similarly, groups in Europe studied a Dutch Red Cross preparation and presented evidence in an open-label study that this material could be used to terminate attacks [45]. Behring Germany prepared C1 inhibitor as a commercial product for treatment of these patients. This material has been on the market for over 25 years and is used extensively in many European countries. The experience of all investigators is that such material terminates attacks [46]. It was essential that efficacy be shown in a double-blind study, since psychological factors clearly play a role in attack frequency and severity. In 1996, Waytes and colleagues, using a preparation prepared by the Austrian company Immuno, in a double-blind placebo-controlled trial, demonstrated that purified C1 inhibitor terminates attacks and that attack termination is prompt [47]. Thus, it is clear from the weight of experience and evidence that purified C1 inhibitor can be used to terminate attacks of HAE.

The approach to treatment of HAE in various countries has recently been outlined in a number of reports. [48–50].

Purified C1 inhibitor, made available by each of two pharmaceutical companies, Lev and ZLB Behring, is currently in clinical trials in the United States as a drug for terminating attacks. As discussed in other chapters, currently there are several other therapies under study. The Dutch company, Pharming, is testing the usefulness of a recombinant human C1 inhibitor made by introducing the human gene into rabbits in such a way that it is secreted into the milk. Attacks of HAE appear to principally involve the kinin generating system and a peptide that inhibits kallikrein, the enzyme that generates bradykinin from high-molecular-weight kininogen (DX88) and a bradykinin receptor type 2 antagonist (Icatibant) are both in clinical trials. Early word from all of the manufacturers suggests that these therapies are successful.

In one generation, we have gone from the complete clinical description of HAE to a description of the gene defect, the characterization of the gene, the understanding of the molecular defects that lead to HAE, and to a great extent an understanding of the pathophysiology of this disease. We have gone from no therapy, to the development of very effective empiric therapy, to the development of much more specific therapy based on pathophysiologic understanding. Although experiments to replace or correct the gene defect in patients with HAE have not been attempted, that is the only step left in developing a complete cure of this illness. Patients have gone from a life-threatening situation to a situation where they can be assured that in the future, their lives will be far more comfortable and productive.

References

[1] Graves R. Clinical lectures on the practice of medicine, 1843. In: Major MH, editor. Classic descriptions of disease. 3rd ed. Springfield, IL: Charles C. Thomas; 1955. p. 623–4.
[2] Quincke H. Concerning the acute localized oedema of the skin. Monatsh. Prakt. Dermat 1882;I:129–31.
[3] Osler W. Hereditary angio-neurotic oedema. Am J Med Sci 1888;95:362–7.
[4] Frank MM, Gelfand JA, Atkinson JP. Hereditary angioedema: the clinical syndrome and its management. Ann Intern Med 1976;84:589–93.
[5] Agostoni A, Cicardi M, Cugno M, et al. Angioedema due to angiotensin-converting enzyme inhibitors. Immunopharmacol 1999;44:21–5.
[6] Frank MM. Effect of sex hormones on the complement-related clinical disorder of hereditary angioedema. Arthritis Rheum 1979;22:1295–9.

[7] Blanco del Val A, Sedano Martenez ME, Carrascal Arranz MI, et al. Hereditary angioede-mal with exclusive abdominal presentation. An Pediatr (Barc) 2004;61:346–7.

[8] Landerman NS, Webster ME, Becker EL, et al. Hereditary angioneurotic edema. J Allergy 1962;33:330–41.

[9] Donaldson VH, Evans RR. A biochemical abnormality in hereditary angioneurotic edema. Am J Med 1963;35:37–44.

[10] Rosen FS, Pensky J, Donaldson V, et al. Hereditary angioneurotic edems: two genetic varients. Science 1965;148:957–8.

[11] Donaldson VH, Rosen FS. Action of complement in hereditary angioedema: the role of C'1 esterase. J Clin Invest 1969;43:2204–13.

[12] Strang CJ, Cholin S, Spragg J, et al. Angioedema induced by a peptide derived from comple-ment component C2. J Exp Med 1988;168(5):1685–98.

[13] Donaldson VH, Rosen FS, Bing DH. Role of the second component of complement (C2) and plasmin in kinin release in hereditary angioneurotic edema (H.A.N.E.) plasma. Trans Assoc Am Physicians 1977;90:174–83.

[14] Brickman CM, Frank MM, Kaliner M. Urine-histamine levels in patients with hereditary angioedema (HAE). J Allergy Clin Immunol 1988;82(3 pt 1):403–6.

[15] Brickman CM, Tsokos GC, Balow JE, et al. Immunoregulatory diseases associated with hereditary angioedema: 1. Clinical manifestations of autoimmune disease. J Allergy Clin Immunol 1986;77(5):749–57.

[16] Zuraw BL. Urticaria, angioedema, and autoimmunity. Clin Lab Med 1997;17(3):559–69.

[17] Cicardi M, Zingale LC, Pappalardo E, et al. Autoantibodies and lymphoproliferative diseases in acquired C1-inhibitor deficiencies. Medicine (Baltimore) 2003;82(4):274–81.

[18] Brickman CM, Tsokos GC, Chused TM, et al. Hereditary angioedema. 2. Serologic and cellular abnormalities. J Allergy Clin Immunol 1986;77(5):758–67.

[19] Spaulding WB. Methyltestosterone therapy for hereditary episodic edema (hereditary angio-neurotic edema). Ann Intern Med 1960;53:739–45.

[20] Gelfand JA, Sherins RJ, Alling DW, et al. Treatment of hereditary angioedema with dana-zol. N Engl J Med 1976;295:1444–8.

[21] Davis PJ, Davis FB, Charache P. Long-term therapy of hereditary angioedema (HAE). Preventive management with fluoxymesterone and oxymetholone in severely affected males and females. Johns Hopkins Med J 1974;135(6):391–8.

[22] Rosse WF, Logue GL, Silberman JR, et al. The effect of synthetic androgens in hereditary angioneurotic edema: alteration of C1 inhibitor and C4 levels. Trans Assoc Am Phys 1976;89:122–32.

[23] Sheffer AL, Fearon DT, Austen KF. Clinical and biochemical effects of stanozolol therapy for hereditary angioedema. J Allergy Clin Immunol 1981;68(3):181–7.

[24] Lappin DF, McPhaden AR, Yap PL, et al. Monocyte C1-inhibitor synthesis in patients with C1-inhibitor deficiency. Eur J Clin Invest 1989;19:45–52.

[25] Pappalardo E, Zingale LC, Cicardi M. Increased expression of C1 inhibitor mRNA in patients with hereditary angioedema treated with danazol. Immunol Lett 2003;86:271–6.

[26] Kang HR, Yim EY, Oh SY, et al. Normal C1 inhibitor mRNA expression level in type 1 hereditary angioedema patients: newly found C1 inhibitor gene mutations. Allergy 2006; 61:260–4.

[27] Hosea SW, Santaella ML, Brown EJ, et al. Long-term therapy of hereditary angioedema with danazol. Ann Intern Med 1980;93(6):809–12.

[28] Zurlo JJ, Frank MM. The long-term safety of danazol in women with hereditary angioede-ma. Fertil Steril 1990;54:64–72.

[29] Cicardi M, Castelli R, Zingale LC, et al. Side effects of long-term prophylaxis with attenu-ated androgens in hereditary angioedema: comparison of treated and untreated patients. J Allergy Clin Immunol 1997;99(2):194–6.

[30] Szeplaki G, Varga L, Valentin S, et al. Adverse effects of danazol prophylaxis on the lipid profiles of patients with hereditary angioedema. J Allergy Clin Immunol 2005;115:864–9.

[31] Church JA. Oxandrolone treatment of childhood hereditary angioedema. Ann Allergy Asthma Immunol 2004;92:377–8.

[32] Nilsson IM, Andersson L, Björkman SE. Epsilon amino-caproic acid (E-ACA) as a therapeutic agent based on 5 years' clinical experience. Acta Med Scand Suppl 1966;448:1–46.

[33] Lundh B, Laurell A-B, Wetterqvist H, et al. A case of hereditary angioneurotic edema successfully treated with epsilon-aminocaproic acid: studies on C'1 esterase inhibitor, C'1 activation, plasminogen level and histamine metabolism. Clin Exp Immunol 1968;3:733–45.

[34] Champion RH, Lachmann PJ. Hereditary angio-oedema treated with epsilon aminocaproic acid. Br J Dermatol 1969;81:763–5.

[35] Frank MM, Sergent JS, Kane MA, et al. Epsilon aminocaproic acid therapy of hereditary angioneurotic edema. A double-blind study. N Engl J Med 1972;286:808–12.

[36] Sheffer AL, Austen KF, Rosen FS. Tranexamic acid therapy in hereditary angioneurotic edema. N Engl J Med 1972;287(9):452–4.

[37] Levi M, Choi G, Picavet C, et al. Self-administration of C1-inhibitor concentrate in patients with hereditary or acquired angioedema caused by C1-inhibitor deficiency. J Allergy Clin Immunol 2006;117(4):904–8.

[38] Jaffe CJ, Atkinson JP, Gelfand JA, et al. Hereditary angioedema: the use of fresh frozen plasma for prophylaxis in patients undergoing oral surgery. J Allergy Clin Immunol 1975; 55:386–93.

[39] Wall RT, Frank MM, Hahn M. A review of 25 patients with hereditary angioedema requiring surgery (see comments). Anesthesiology 1989;71(2):309–11.

[40] Atkinson JC, Frank MM. Oral manifestations and dental management of patients with hereditary angioedema. J Oral Pathol Med 1991;20(3):139–42.

[41] Sheffer AL, Fearon DT, Austen KF, et al. Tranexamic acid: preoperative prophylactic therapy for patients with hereditary angioneurotic edema. J Allergy Clin Immunol 1977;60(1): 38–40.

[42] Farkas H, Gyeney L, Gidofalvy E, et al. The efficacy of short-term danazol prophylaxis in hereditary angioedema patients undergoing maxillofacial and dental procedures. J Oral Maxillofac Surg 1999;57(4):404–8.

[43] Pickering RJ, Good RA, Kelly JR, et al. Replacement therapy in hereditary angioedema. Successful treatment of two patients with fresh frozen plasma. Lancet 1969;1(7590):326–30.

[44] Gadek JE, Hosea SW, Gelfand JA, et al. Replacement therapy in hereditary angioedema. N Engl J Med 1980;302:542–6.

[45] Agostoni A, Bergamaschini L, Martignoni G, et al. Treatment of acute attacks of hereditary angioedema with C1-inhibitor concentrate. Ann Allergy 1980;44(5):299–301.

[46] Bork K, Meng G, Staubach P, et al. Hereditary angioedema: new findings concerning symptoms, affected organs, and course. Am J Med 2006;119:267–74.

[47] Waytes AT, Rosen FS, Frank MM. Treatment of hereditary angioedema with a vapor-heated C1 inhibitor concentrate. N Engl J Med 1996;334(25):1630–4.

[48] Bowen B, Hawk JJ, Sibunka S, et al. A review of the reported defects in the human C1 exterase inhibitor gene producing hereditary angioedema including four new mutations. Clin Immunol 2001;98:157–63.

[49] Gompels MM, Lock RJ, Abinun M, et al. C1 inhibitor deficiency: consensus document. Clin Exp Immunol 2005;139:379–94.

[50] Farkas H. Hereditary and acquired angioedema: problems and progress: proceedings of the third C1 esterase inhibitor deficiency workshop and beyond. J Allergy Clin Immunol 2004;114(Suppl 3):S51–131.

ELSEVIER
SAUNDERS

Immunol Allergy Clin N Am
26 (2006) 669–690

IMMUNOLOGY
AND ALLERGY
CLINICS
OF NORTH AMERICA

Acquired Deficiency of the Inhibitor of the First Complement Component: Presentation, Diagnosis, Course, and Conventional Management

Lorenza Chiara Zingale, MD[a], Roberto Castelli, MD[b],
Andrea Zanichelli, MD[a], Marco Cicardi, MD[a],*

[a]*Department of Internal Medicine, San Giuseppe Hospital—AFaR (Ospedale San Giuseppe), University of Milan, Via San Vittore 12, 20123 Milano, Italy*
[b]*Department of Internal Medicine, IRCCS Fondazione Ospedale Maggiore Policlinico, Via Pace 9, 20122 Milano, Italy*

Acquired first complement component inhibitor deficiency is a rare syndrome characterized by consumption of the inhibitor of the first complement component (C1-INH) and hyperactivation of the classic complement pathway. The condition is frequently referred in the literature as "acquired angioedema," but this term could generate confusion with other forms of nonhereditary angioedema characterized by normal C1-INH; hence, the authors prefer not to use it and to refer to this condition as angioedema with acquired C1-INH deficiency.

Caldwell and colleagues [1] described the first patient in 1972. Since that time, several other cases have been reported, mostly associated with lymphoproliferative disorders. In 1986, Jackson and colleagues [2] discovered an autoreactive immunoglobulin G against C1-INH in a patient who had angioedema and acquired C1-INH deficiency. This finding demonstrated that an autoimmune mechanism could be the cause of acquired C1-INH deficiency. The relationship between lymphoproliferative-related and autoimmune C1-INH deficiency has been and continues to be a matter of debate, reflecting the uncertainty in defining the etiopathogenesis of this condition (Fig. 1).

* Corresponding author.
E-mail address: marco.cicardi@unimi.it (M. Cicardi).

0889-8561/06/$ - see front matter © 2006 Elsevier Inc. All rights reserved.
doi:10.1016/j.iac.2006.08.002   *immunology.theclinics.com*

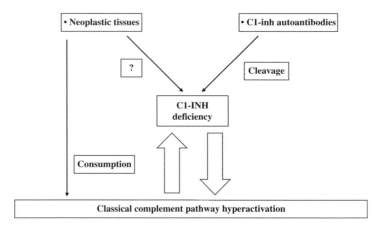

Fig. 1. Pathogenetic mechanisms in acquired C1-INH deficiency.

Etiopathogenesis

Several attempts have been made to clarify the mechanism responsible for the consumption of C1-INH and for the massive activation of the classic complement pathway. Here the authors summarize the most important steps in the understanding of this etiopathogenetic puzzle.

Initial experiments explored the hypothesis that C1-INH or the classic complement pathway was consumed by the neoplastic lymphatic tissues, and in several patients this hypothesis could be confirmed [1,3,4]. Further understanding of the mechanism of complement consumption came from Geha and colleagues [5], who demonstrated the possibility that some patients who had acquired C1-INH deficiency and paraproteins had immunoglobulins against the idiotypic determinants of the M components. These idiotype–anti-idiotype immune complexes fixed C1q and consumed C1-INH. However, this finding has not been confirmed in subsequent patients. Direct proof that patients who had acquired C1-INH deficiency had in vivo increased consumption of C1-INH was provided in 1986 by Melamed and colleagues [6], who injected patients with radiolabeled C1-INH and C1q.

In 1986, Jackson and colleagues [2] demonstrated the presence of an autoreactive immunoglobulin G against C1-INH in a patient who had acquired C1 inhibitor deficiency. Because the first patients who had autoantibodies to C1-INH looked otherwise healthy [2,7], acquired C1-INH deficiency was divided into two separate forms: type I, paraneoplastic, mainly associated with lymphatic malignancies or other diseases; and type II, autoimmune, caused by autoantibodies to C1-INH. This separation was later questioned because the two conditions coexisted in several patients [8–10].

The evidence for an autoantibody-mediated C1-INH deficiency raises two important questions: (1) What is the mechanism used by the autoantibody to deplete C1-INH? (2) What is the underlying disorder in lymphocyte maturation that leads to the expansion of the autoreactive lymphocytes? The first of these questions has been addressed by several experimental approaches. Studies in monocytes from a patient who had the so-called "autoimmune" C1-INH deficiency demonstrated that these cells secreted structurally and functionally normal C1-INH, which was then consumed by the autoantibodies [11]. The majority of these autoantibodies bind epitopes around the reactive center of C1-INH [12–14]. By this binding they destabilize the C1-INH–protease complex or enhance susceptibility of C1-INH to proteolytic cleavage (see article elsewhere in this issue). In fact, a large quantity of cleaved inactive C1-INH circulates in the serum of most patients who have acquired C1-INH deficiency and autoantibodies to C1-INH [7,11,15–18]. The cleavage appears to be primarily dependent on the activated contact system, as suggested by Zuraw and colleagues [19], who first described cleaved C1-INH in patients who had acquired deficiency. Accordingly, when C1-INH activity increases in patients who have autoantibodies, there is a reduction in both the cleaved form of C1-INH and the signs of contact system activation [16,20]. Together, these results elucidate the mechanism used by the autoantibodies to consume C1-INH, but they leave unexplained the mechanism leading to tremendous classic pathway activation and C1 consumption, which characterize acquired C1-INH deficiency. Indeed, by depleting C1-INH, autoantibodies create a condition similar to that of hereditary C1-INH deficiency, with additional massive consumption of C1. It is possible, however, that additional, still unknown factors could intervene to enhance classic pathway complement activation.

The attempt to unravel the causes of the expansion of anti–C1-INH autoreactive B lymphocyte clones offers the possibility of seeing acquired C1-INH deficiency, whether associated with autoantibodies or with B cell proliferation, within the same scenario. Several lines of evidence suggest that autoreactive and neoplastic lymphoproliferation share part of the molecular mechanism that facilitates expansion of deviating clones [21]. Paraproteins from different conditions may bind autoantigens [22]. It has been shown that the associations between certain autoimmune disorders and the risk for non-Hodgkin lymphoma (NHL) may be not general but rather mediated through specific NHL subtypes. These NHL subtypes develop during postantigen exposure stages of lymphocyte differentiation, consistent with a role for antigenic drive in autoimmunity-related lymphoma genesis [23]. Thus, we may speculate that all acquired C1-INH deficiencies may depend on proliferation of clones recognizing C1-INH. These clones may subsequently expand with characteristics of autoimmune or neoplastic proliferation. Experimental proof of this hypothesis needs to be provided.

Lymphoproliferative diseases and acquired first complement component inhibitor deficiencies

Reviewing the literature, the authors recorded 136 patients who had angioedema and acquired C1-INH deficiency. The characteristics of these patients are detailed in Table 1. Many of them had various forms of B cell lymphoproliferative diseases that ranged from monoclonal gammopathies of undetermined significance (MGUS) to true malignancies [3,8,24–28]. In 27 patients (one out of five), NHL was diagnosed. Taking into account that the prevalence of NHL is 114 per 100,000 inhabitants, according to data from the collaborative study of the Italian cancer registry, it is clear that the risk for NHL is markedly increased in patients who have angioedema and acquired C1-INH deficiency. Analyzing these cases of NHL according to the revised European-American lymphoma (REAL) classification, the authors find that five were of high-grade malignancy (one large B cell lymphoma, two mantle cell lymphomas, one lymphosarcoma, one immunoblastic lymphoma), and 14 were indolent NHL (six small lymphocytic lymphomas, four marginal zone lymphomas, four cases of lymphoplasmacytoid lymphoma/Waldeström disease). Follicular lymphoma, the most frequent histotype of indolent NHL, has never been reported in association with acquired C1-INH deficiency; this finding is in agreement with the other series of patients who had autoimmune disease and indolent NHL [23,29]. In the remaining eight patients, the histologic pattern was not reported, or it was not in agreement with the REAL classification.

Forty-seven of 136 patients (34.5%) who had angioedema and acquired C1-INH deficiency fulfilled the diagnostic criteria for MGUS (ie, serum monoclonal protein level less than 3 g/dL or less than 2 g/dL for IgA, less than 10% plasma cells in bone marrow and absence of lytic bone lesions, anemia, hypercalcemia, and renal failure). Given that the prevalence of MGUS in the general population younger than 70 years is approximately 3%, prevalence of this condition is definitely increased in angioedema with acquired C1-INH deficiency. However, based on a study from the authors' group, patients who have angioedema due to acquired C1-INH deficiency and MGUS have no additional risk for myeloma progression as compared with the general population [8]. The authors also found that, when MGUS and autoantibodies to C1-INH coexist, they frequently share the same heavy and light chain isotypes. Characterization of the electrophoretic mobility of the two immunoglobulins is strongly in favor of their identity and suggests that the monoclonal component derives from the clonal expansion of anti–C1-INH autoantibody-producing cells [16].

Presentation

The typical symptom of C1 inhibitor deficiency, whether hereditary or acquired, is angioedema [30]: a recurrent, self-limiting, nonpitting, nonpruritic edema that completely resolves in 1 to 5 days without any local or systemic damage. Like hereditary angioedema, the angioedema associated with acquired C1-INH deficiency affects primarily three sites: the subcutaneous tissue, the gastrointestinal mucosa, and the mucosa of the upper respiratory tract. Angioedema of the skin causes deformities, which may involve the face, genitals, buttocks, and extremities with no particular preference. Urticaria is usually absent, although transient and mild urticarial eruptions (erythema marginatum) may herald the overt swelling. Cutaneous angioedema creates discomfort in the patient: it can impair social life if it deforms the face or affects the function of hands and feet. Abdominal attacks are characterized by vomiting, colicky abdominal pain, and, more rarely, by diarrhea. These symptoms usually subside spontaneously within 2 days if not treated. Dysphagia, voice change, and respiratory stridor are signs of involvement of upper airways and may precede asphyxia due to laryngeal edema. This condition is life-threatening and requires immediate emergency therapy. In the past it was the principal case of death in C1-INH–deficient patients.

Diagnosis

The clinical presentation is similar to that of hereditary C1-INH deficiency. The differences between the two forms are absence of family history, late onset of symptoms (after the fourth decade of life), and response to treatment [8]. Clinical suspicion should be confirmed by laboratory analysis. The typical biochemical picture of acquired C1-INH deficiency is the following: C1-INH function and antigen, C4 and C1q markedly reduced (usually far below 50% of normal), with a normal C3. Nonetheless, variations on this picture have been reported. C1-INH antigen can be normal, when elevated amounts of cleaved inactive C1-INH circulate in plasma. A minority of patients have normal C1q. In rare instances at the onset of the disease, C1-INH function tends to return to normal between angioedema attacks.

Any patient who has acquired C1 inhibitor deficiency should be tested for autoantibodies to C1-INH. Autoantibodies to C1-INH may be detected as immunoglobulins preventing C1-INH function or binding C1-INH. In the first assay, immunoglobulins isolated from serum block the activity of C1-INH, measured as inhibition of conversion of synthetic substrates specific for its target proteases [31]. In 1987, Alsenz and colleagues [7] developed a solid-phase ELISA for detecting immunoglobulins binding to C1-INH coated to microtiter plates. This simple and highly sensitive method is still used with slight modifications [8,28].

Course

The course of and prognosis for angioedema with acquired C1-INH deficiency depend on the underlying disease and the availability of proper therapy for life-threatening angioedema. Although angioedema attacks usually resolve without treatment, patients are exposed to the risk for laryngeal edema. In such an emergency, substitutive therapy with plasma-derived C1-INH remains so far the only treatment with a consistent likelihood of success, the alternative being emergency tracheostomy. The uneven

Table 1
Literature on acquired first complement component inhibitor deficiency

	Reference	Associated disease	Chemo therapy	αC1-INH	M comp	Time lag AE/A. Dis	Follow-up	Cause of death
B cell neoplasms								
1.	Bouillet, et al, 2000 [33]	IgA myeloma	Yes	No	IgA	0 y	?	...
2.	Sheffer, et al, 1985 [38]	IgA myeloma	No	ND	IgA	2 y	2 y	...
3.	Gordon, et al, 1983 [81]	IgG myeloma	Yes	ND	IgG	...	50 y	...
4.	Schreiber, et al, 1976 [3]	Immunoblastic lymphoma	Yes	ND	IgM	0 y	1 y	Pneumonia
5.	Bohle, et al, 1996 [80]	Immunocytoma/ Colon K	Yes/Splenectomy	ND	IgM	...	11 y	...
6.	Bohle, et al, 1996 [80]	Immunocytoma/ Hodgkin disease	Yes/Splenectomy	ND	IgM	1 y	5 y	...
7.	Cicardi, et al, 2003 [8]	Large B cell lymphoma	Yes	None	No	...	12 y	...
8.	Cicardi, et al, 2003 [8]	LNH low grade	Yes	None	None	...	1 y	...
9.	Bouillet, et al, 2000 [33]	Low-grade NHL	Yes	No	No	2 y	3 y	...
10.	Fremeaux-Bacchi, et al, 2002 [28]	Low-grade NHL	...	Yes	IgAλ	...	...	...
11.	Beretta, et al, 1991 [85]	Low-grade NHL	No	No	No	−1 y	0.5 y	...
12.	Markovic, et al, 2000 [54]	Low-grade NHL	Yes	ND	No	2 y	2 y	...
13.	Fiechtner, et al, 1980 [79]	Lymphoblastic lymphoma	Yes	ND	No	3 y	6 y	...

14.	Richardson, et al, 1989 [78]	Lymphocytic lymphoma	Yes	ND	No	2 y	6 y	...
15.	Rosenfeld, et al, 1975 [77]	Lymphocytic lymphoma	?	ND	IgM	...	...	...
16.	Cicardi, et al, 2003 [8]	Lymphocytic lymphoma	Yes	No	No	...	3 y	...
17.	Sheffer, et al, 1985 [38]	Lymphocytic NHL	No	ND	No	3 y	3 y	...
18.	Gottlieb, et al, 1983 [62]	Lymphoma	...	...	...	...	...	...
19.	Cicardi, et al, 2003 [8]	Lymphoplasmocytic lymphoma	Yes	IgGk	IgMk	...	9 y	...
20.	Hauptmann, et al, 1977 [76]	Lymphoproliferative disorder	Yes	ND	IgM	...	6 mo	...
21.	Caldwell, et al, 1972 [1]	Lymphosarcoma	Splenectomy	ND	No	1.5 y	6 y	Seizures
22.	Sheffer, et al, 1985 [38]	Anapl lymphocytic lymphoma	Yes	ND	No	1.5 y	4 y	Sepsis
23.	Chevrant-Breton, et al, 1982 [82]	CLL	No	ND	No	2 y	>4 y	...
24.	Day, et al, 1976 [83]	CLL	?	ND	?	...	...	...
25.	Dreyfus, et al, 1981 [34]	CLL	Yes	ND	IgM	0 y (?)	18 mo	...
26.	Dreyfus, et al, 1981 [34]	CLL	Yes	ND	No	–6 y	10 y	...
27.	Lafeuillade, et al, 1993 [86]	CLL	Yes	No	No	–0.5 y	1 y	...
28.	Lipscombe, et al, 1996 [67]	CLL	No	ND	No	–7 y	10	...

(continued on next page)

Table 1 (continued)

	Reference	Associated disease	Chemo therapy	αC1-INH	M comp	Time lag AE/A. Dis	Follow-up	Cause of death
29.	Postlethwaite, et al, 1988 [61]	CLL	Yes	...	IgM	0 y	?	...
30.	Sheffer, et al, 1985 [38]	CLL	Yes	ND	No	3 y	5 y	...
31.	Sheffer, et al, 1985 [38]	CLL	Yes	ND	No	−2 y	3.5 y	Peritonitis
32.	Chevailler, et al, 1996 [24]	CLL/ Lymphoplasmacytic lymphoma	Yes	IgA	IgM/A	−1 y	14 y	Pneumonia
33.	Bouillet, et al, 2000 [33]	Heavy chain disease	Yes	No	Yes	0 y	?	...
34.	Shahar, et al, 1997 [60]	Mantle cell lymphoma/ Myeloma	Splenectomy	...	...	...	...	...
35.	Markovic, et al, 2000 [54]	Mantle-cell lymphoma	No	ND	No	0 y	5 mo	...
36.	Frigas, 1989 [65]	Small cleaved-cell lymphoma	No	ND	No	1 y	1 y	...
37.	Bain, et al, 1993 [27]	Small lymphocytic lymphoma	No	ND	IgM	8 y	6 y	...
38.	Bain, et al, 1993 [27]	Splenic lymphoma with villous lymphocytes	Yes	ND	No	0.5 y	2 y	...
39.	Bain, et al, 1993 [27]	Splenic lymphoma with villous lymphocytes	Yes	ND	IgM	3 y	8 y	...
40.	Gaur, et al, 2004 [84]	Splenic marginal zone lymphoma	Splenectomy	ND	IgM	0	5 y	1
41.	Fremeaux-Bacchi, et al, 2002 [28]	Splenic NHL	...	Yes	IgMλ	...	...	...
42.	Casali, et al, 1978 [41]	W macroglobulinemia	?	ND	IgM	?	?	...

43.	Delmer, et al, 1993 [73]	W macroglobulinemia	Yes	ND	IgM	2 y	3 y	...
44.	Baldwin, et al, 1991 [75]	NHL	No	ND	No	1.5 y	2 y	...
45.	Mathur, et al, 1993 [26]	NHL	?	ND	IgM	...	...	...
46.	Rodriguez, et al, 1988 [74]	NHL	Yes	ND	No	0.5 y	1 y	...
47.	Cicardi, et al, 2003 [8]	Marginal zone cell lymphoma	Yes	IgM	...	...	8 y	...
Monoclonal gammopathies of undetermined significance (MGUS)								
48.	Bouillet, et al, 2000 [33]	MGUS	No	IgG	IgG	...	?	...
49.	Bouillet, et al, 2000 [33]	MGUS	No	IgG	IgM/G	...	>10 mo	...
50.	Bouillet, et al, 2000 [33]	MGUS	No	IgM	IgM	...	?	...
51.	Bouillet, et al, 2000 [33]	MGUS	No	No	Yes	0 y	?	...
52.	Boyar, et al, 1993 [64]	MGUS	No	IgG/A	IgG	...	5 y	...
53.	Chevailler, et al, 1996 [24]	MGUS	No	IgA	IgA	...	5 y	...
54.	Chevailler, et al, 1996 [24]	MGUS	No	IgG/M	IgM	...	1 y	Laryngeal edema
55.	Cicardi, et al, 2003 [8]	MGUS	No	IgMkλ	IgMk	0 y	11 y	...
56.	Cicardi, et al, 2003 [8]	MGUS	No	IgGλ	IgGλ	...	8 y	...

(continued on next page)

Table 1 (continued)

	Reference	Associated disease	Chemo therapy	αC1-INH	M comp	Time lag AE/A. Dis	Follow-up	Cause of death
57.	Cicardi, et al, 2003 [8]	MGUS	No	IgM/ IgGλ	IgGλ	...	5 y	...
58.	Cicardi, et al, 2003 [8]	MGUS	No	IgAλ	IgGλ	...	6 y	...
59.	Cicardi, et al, 2003 [8]	MGUS	No	IgGK	IgGK	...	13 y	...
60.	Cicardi, et al, 2003 [8]	MGUS	No	IgMk	IgMk	...	1 y	...
61.	Cicardi, et al, 2003 [8]	MGUS	No	None	IgGK	...	6 y	...
62.	Cicardi, et al, 2003 [8]	MGUS	No	None	IgGλ	...	2 y	...
63.	Cicardi, et al, 2003 [8]	MGUS	No	None	IgGλ	...	1 y	...
64.	Cicardi, et al, 2003 [8]	MGUS	No	IgAλ	IgAλ	...	11 y	...
65.	Cicardi, et al, 2003 [8]	MGUS	No	IgMλ	IgMλ	...	24 y	...
66.	Fremeaux-Bacchi, et al, 2002 [28]	MGUS	...	Yes	IgAk	...	...	...
67.	Fremeaux-Bacchi, et al, 2002 [28]	MGUS	...	Yes	IgAk	...	...	...
68.	Fremeaux-Bacchi, et al, 2002 [28]	MGUS	...	Yes	IgAλ	...	...	...
69.	Fremeaux-Bacchi, et al, 2002 [28]	MGUS	No	Yes	IgGk	...	...	...
70.	Fremeaux-Bacchi, et al, 2002 [28]	MGUS	No	Yes	IgGk	...	...	...

(continued on next page)

71.	Fremeaux-Bacchi, et al, 2002 [28]	MGUS	No	Yes	IgGk	...	...	...	...
72.	Fremeaux-Bacchi, et al, 2002 [28]	MGUS	No	Yes	IgGk	...	...	...	...
73.	Fremeaux-Bacchi, et al, 2002 [28]	MGUS	No	Yes	IgGk	...	...	...	...
74.	Fremeaux-Bacchi, et al, 2002 [28]	MGUS	No	Yes	IgGk	...	...	...	...
75.	Fremeaux-Bacchi, et al, 2002 [28]	MGUS	No	Yes	IgGk	...	...	...	...
76.	Fremeaux-Bacchi, et al, 2002 [28]	MGUS	No	Yes	IgMk	...	...	...	...
77.	Fremeaux-Bacchi, et al, 2002 [28]	MGUS	No	Yes	IgMk	...	...	...	...
78.	Fremeaux-Bacchi, et al, 2002 [28]	MGUS	No	Yes	IgMk	...	...	...	...
79.	Fremeaux-Bacchi, et al, 2002 [28]	MGUS	No	Yes	IgMk	...	...	...	...
80.	Fremeaux-Bacchi, et al, 2002 [28]	MGUS	No	Yes	IgMk	...	...	...	...
81.	Fremeaux-Bacchi, et al, 2002 [28]	MGUS	No	Yes	IgMk	...	...	...	...
82.	Frigas, 1989 [65]	MGUS	No	ND	IgG	...	7 y	...	...
83.	He, et al, 1996 #128 [14]	MGUS	No	IgG	IgG	...	?	...	...
84.	He, et al, 1996 #128 [14]	MGUS	No	IgG	IgG	...	?	...	...
85.	He, et al, 1996 [14]	MGUS	No	IgG	IgG	...	?	...	...
86.	Hentges, et al, 1986 [66]	MGUS	No	ND	IgG	...	6 y	...	...

Table 1 (*continued*)

	Reference	Associated disease	Chemo therapy	αC1-INH	M comp	Time lag AE/A. Dis	Follow-up	Cause of death
87.	Kleiner, et al, 2001 [70]	MGUS	No	IgG	IgG	…	…	…
88.	Lipscombe, et al, 1996 [67]	MGUS	No	ND	IgM	…	…	…
89.	Malbran, et al, 1988 [17]	MGUS	No	IgA	Yes	…	12 y	…
90.	Malbran, et al, 1988 [17]	MGUS	No	IgA	Yes	…	17 y	…
91.	Malbran, et al, 1988 [17]	MGUS	No	IgG	Yes	…	1 y	…
92.	Malcolm, et al, 1999 [68]	MGUS	No	ND	Yes	…	3 y	…
93.	Sinclair, et al, 2004 [69].	MGUS	No	ND	IgG	…	…	3
94.	Cicardi, et al, 2003 [8]	MGUS hydatidosis	No	IgGK	IgGK	…	24 y	…
Auto-immune disease								
95.	Hauptmann, et al, 1976 [25]	AIHA	Yes	ND	IgM	…	6 mo	…
96.	Mandle, et al, 1994 [12]	Cryoglobulinemia	No	Igk	No	…	?	…
97.	Casali, et al, 1978 [41]	Essential cryoglobulinemia	?	ND	IgM	…	?	…
98.	Fremeaux-Bacchi, et al, 2002 [28]	RA	…	Yes	…	…	…	…
99.	Cacoub, et al, 2001 [92]	SLE	…	No	…	…	…	…
100.	Cacoub, et al, 2001 [92]	SLE	…	No	…	…	…	…

	Reference	Condition						
101.	Cacoub, et al, 2001 [92]	SLE	...	No	...	...	...	...
102.	Ochonisky, et al, 1993 [87]	SLE	No	No	No	2 y	9 y	...
Other neoplasms								
103.	Fremeaux-Bacchi, et al, 2002 [28]	Adenoca gastric	...	Yes	...	...	...	...
104.	Wasserfallen, et al, 1995 [39]	Adenocarcinoma (linitis plastica)	Surgery	ND	No	0.5 y	2 y	Cachessia
105.	Cohen, et al, 1978 [32]	Adenocarcinoma of rectum	Surgery	ND	No	1 y	3 y	...
106.	Cicardi, et al, 2003 [8]	Breast cancer	Yes	IgAλ	...	...	12 y	...
107.	Alonso, et al, 2002 [91]	Ca bladder	...	ND	...	...	...	...
108.	Fremeaux-Bacchi, et al, 2002 [28]	Ca colon	...	Yes	...	...	...	...
109.	Fremeaux-Bacchi, et al, 2002 [28]	Ca pancreas	...	Yes	...	...	...	...
110.	van Spronsen, et al, 1998 [63]	Malignant hypernephroma	No	IgA	IgA	1 y	9 y	...
Other diseases								
111.	Chadenat, 2000 [96]	Echinococcus granulosus	No	IgG	No	...	3 y	...
112.	Spath, et al, 1989 [71]	Fibroleiomyoma of uterus	No	IgG	No	3 y	3 y	...
113.	Farkas, et al, 1999 [88]	Helicobacter pylori	...	No	No	...	...	...
114.	Fremeaux-Bacchi, et al, 2002 [28]	Hydatidosis	...	Yes	...	...	...	...

(continued on next page)

Table 1 (*continued*)

	Reference	Associated disease	Chemo therapy	αC1-INH	M comp	Time lag AE/A. Dis	Follow-up	Cause of death
115.	Nilsen, et al, 1980 [36]	Myelofibrosis	No	ND	No	1 y	5 mo	...
116.	Wautier, et al, 1981 [94]	Thrombotic disorders	...	...	...	...	...	...
117.	Wautier, et al, 1981 [94]	Thrombotic disorders	...	...	...	...	...	...
118.	Széplaki, et al, 2006 [93]	Thrombofilia	...	IgG/A	...	...	50 mo	...
No disease								
119.	Alsenz, et al, 1987 [7]	None	No	IgG	No	...	2 y	...
120.	Alsenz, et al, 1987 [7]	None	No	IgG	No	...	5 y	...
121.	Bouillet, et al, 2000 [33]	None	No	IgG	No	...	?	...
122.	Cicardi, et al, 2003 [8]	None	No	IgAK	No	...	8 y	...
123.	Cicardi, et al, 2003 [8]	None	No	IgG	No	...	1 y	...
124.	Cicardi, et al, 2003 [8]	None	No	IgGK	No	...	1 y	...
125.	Cicardi, et al, 2003 [8]	None	No	IgMλ	No	...	5 y	...
126.	Donaldson, et al, 1992 [18]	None	...	IgG	No	...	8 y	...
127.	Fremeaux-Bacchi, et al, 2002 [28]	None	...	Yes	...	...	...	...
128.	Fremeaux-Bacchi, et al, 2002 [28]	None	...	Yes	...	...	...	...

129. He, et al, 1996 [14]	None	No	IgM	No	?	...
130. He, et al, 1996 [14]	None	No	IgM	No	?	...
131. He, et al, 1996 [14]	None	No	IgM	No	?	...
132. Higa, et al, 2002 [90]	None	Yes	...	...	...	...
133. Jackson, et al, 1986 [2]	None	No	IgG	No	?	...
134. Ponce, et al, 2002 [89]	None	No	IgG/M	...	...	...
135. Valsecchi, et al, 1997 [72]	None	No	IgM	...	55 mo	...
136. Zuraw, et al, 1991 [20]	None	No	IgG/A	No	3 y	...

B cell neoplasm 47

MGUS 47
Autoimmune disease 8
Other neoplasms 8
Other diseases 8
No disease 18
Total 136

Abbreviations: AE/A. Dis, angioedema/associated disease; AIHA, autoimmune hemolytic anemia; Anapl, anaplastic; Ca, carcinoma; CLL, chronic lymphocytic leukemia; k, immunoglobin light chain k; LNH, non-Hodgkin lymphoma; M Comp, monoclonal component; ND, not done; RA, rheumatoid arthritis; SLE₁, systemic lupus erythematosus; W, Waldenström; αC1-INH, anti C1-INH autoantibody.

availability of this treatment in different countries (eg, it is not approved in the United States) creates important differences in the standard of care. Even though official epidemiologic data are not available, the risk for death from C1-INH deficiency appears to be higher when plasma-derived C1-INH is not readily accessible.

Successful treatment of the underlying disease has been shown to resolve angioedema symptoms and biochemical abnormalities in patients who have acquired C1-INH deficiency. The first such report from Cohen and colleagues [32] has been repeatedly confirmed [4,8,27,33–39], although the details of the responses have demonstrated a wide range of variability. Disappearance of angioedema may be temporary, even without evidence of a relapse of the associated disease [32,35]. In other patients [8], however, symptoms and complement parameters reverted to normal on remission of the associated lymphoproliferative disease and did not return even on recurrence of the malignancy. Conversely, patients may continue with unchanged biochemical abnormalities but cease completely to have symptoms of angioedema.

The authors reported one patient [8] who experienced severe angioedema symptoms for 5 years that ended abruptly, independently of any treatment or other apparent reason. Despite the clinical remission, his C1-INH remained low until he died 18 years later from complications of hepatitis C, without further angioedema. Another patient [40] began to have angioedema after an echinococcal cyst was removed from her liver. Seven years later she underwent a second surgery for relapse of the echinococcal cyst. After the second surgery, the patient experienced a transient normalization of C1-INH that lasted a few weeks before the C1-INH levels again fell. The echinococcus did not recur, and she remained asymptomatic for angioedema until she died 20 years later from unrelated causes. Other cases of patients who had no symptoms of angioedema despite a persistent C1-INH deficiency are documented in the literature [1,34,41–44].

Based on all these different situations, the authors conclude that the relationship between angioedema, C1-INH deficiency, and associated disease is still unclear, rendering the outcome for patients unpredictable.

Conventional management

Therapy for acquired C1-INH deficiency follows two directions: treatment of the associated diseases and prevention or reversal of angioedema symptoms. As already mentioned, cure of the underlying disease has induced clinical remission of angioedema symptoms. In the past, immunosuppressive regimens (cyclophosphamide, with or without steroids) have been used for suppressing the formation of anti–C1-INH autoantibodies in isolated patients who had acquired C1-INH deficiency [11,18,24,39]. Because of its side effects, the indication for immunosuppression in the absence of malignancy is highly questionable [45], and in the authors' opinion it should be considered only in patients who have severe, intractable recurrences of angioedema.

The management of angioedema in patients who have acquired C1-INH deficiency has been directly derived from that of the hereditary form [46], but the response has not always been the same. In some cases, acquired C1-INH–deficient patients may be resistant to these treatments [15,18,33,44,47].

For long-term prevention of angioedema recurrences, patients are treated with attenuated androgens and antifibrinolytic agents, the same treatments used for many years in hereditary angioedema (HAE) [48–50]. Compared with patients who have HAE, patients who have acquired C1-INH deficiency are often resistant to attenuated androgens [47,51]. By contrast, they show a much better response to antifibrinolytic agents, which are currently the authors' first choice [8]. Antifibrinolytic agents appear to be well tolerated [52], but it is still debatable whether they carry an increased risk for thrombosis. Although this question has not been definitively answered, the authors prefer to institute concomitant oral anticoagulant therapy in patients who have increased risk for thromboembolism and need long-term antifibrinolytic therapy [8].

Long-term prophylaxis with plasma-derived C1-INH has been successfully performed in patients who have acquired C1-INH deficiency using higher doses compared with those used in HAE [53].

The treatment of acute attacks remains a crucial issue for these patients. Despite an isolated indication that conventional antiallergic therapy may have some effect [54], the great majority of physicians actively involved in the diagnosis and treatment of C1-INH deficiency consider this approach unreliable [46,55]. The common experience is that, although angioedema attacks resolve spontaneously, severe attacks may be successfully treated only with the prompt infusion of plasma-derived C1-INH. Several studies confirmed its effectiveness in patients who have hereditary angioedema [56–59]. No controlled study has been performed in patients who have acquired C1-INH deficiency. The reported experiences indicate that this treatment is usually also effective in this condition, although variable degrees of resistance in some patients may necessitate higher doses [15,47,53]. The authors experienced one patient who is a nonresponder because of the rapid C1-INH catabolism [47]. This severe condition calls for the discovery of an alternative to the treatment with plasma-derived C1-INH. New compounds are now being tested in clinical trials to assess their capacity to revert acute attacks in C1-INH–deficient patients. One of them, Dx88 (Dyax Corp., Cambridge, Massachusetts; see article elsewhere in this issue), has been successfully used in an open-label study, also in two patients who had acquired C1 inhibitor deficiency. A recent paper reported the interesting finding that a series of four weekly injections with Rituximab (a chimeric monoclonal antibody to CD20) induced long-lasting remission in angioedema symptoms together with a near normalization of C1-INH and C4 levels in three patients with severe acquired C1-INH deficiency [95].

References

[1] Caldwell JR, Ruddy S, Schur PH, et al. Acquired C1 inhibitor deficiency in lymphosarcoma. Clin Immunol Immunopathol 1972;1:39–52.

[2] Jackson J, Sim RB, Whelan A, et al. An IgG autoantibody which inactivates C1-inhibitor. Nature 1986;323(6090):722–4.

[3] Schreiber AD, Zweiman B, Atkins P, et al. Acquired angioedema with lymphoproliferative disorder: association of C1 inhibitor deficiency with cellular abnormality. Blood 1976;48(4): 567–80.

[4] Hauptmann G, Petitjean F, Lang JM, et al. Acquired C1 inhibitor deficiency in a case of lymphosarcoma of the spleen. Reversal of complement abnormalities after splenectomy. Clin Exp Immunol 1979;37(3):523–31.

[5] Geha RS, Quinti I, Austen KF, et al. Acquired C1-inhibitor deficiency associated with antiidiotypic antibody to monoclonal immunoglobulins. N Engl J Med 1985;312(9): 534–40.

[6] Melamed J, Alper CA, Cicardi M, et al. The metabolism of C1 inhibitor and C1q in patients with acquired C1-inhibitor deficiency. J Allergy Clin Immunol 1986;77(2):322–6.

[7] Alsenz J, Bork K, Loos M. Autoantibody-mediated acquired deficiency of C1 inhibitor. N Engl J Med 1987;316(22):1360–6.

[8] Cicardi M, Zingale LC, Pappalardo E, et al. Autoantibodies and lymphoproliferative diseases in acquired C1-inhibitor deficiencies. Medicine (Baltimore) 2003;82(4):274–81.

[9] D'Incan M, Tridon A, Ponard D, et al. Acquired angioedema with C1 inhibitor deficiency: is the distinction between type I and type II still relevant? Dermatology 1999;199(3): 227–30.

[10] Whaley K, Sim RB, He S. Autoimmune C1-inhibitor deficiency. Clin Exp Immunol 1996; 106(3):423–6.

[11] Jackson J, Sim RB, Whaley K, et al. Autoantibody facilitated cleavage of C1-inhibitor in autoimmune angioedema. J Clin Invest 1989;83(2):698–707.

[12] Mandle R, Baron C, Roux E, et al. Acquired C1 inhibitor deficiency as a result of an autoantibody to the reactive center region of C1 inhibitor. J Immunol 1994;152(9):4680–5.

[13] Donaldson VH, Wagner CJ, Davis AE 3rd. An autoantibody to C1-inhibitor recognizes the reactive center of the inhibitor. J Lab Clin Med 1996;127(2):229–32.

[14] He S, Tsang S, North J, et al. Epitope mapping of C1 inhibitor autoantibodies from patients with acquired C1 inhibitor deficiency. J Immunol 1996;156(5):2009–13.

[15] Alsenz J, Lambris JD, Bork K, et al. Acquired C1 inhibitor (C1-INH) deficiency type II. Replacement therapy with C1-INH and analysis of patients' C1-INH and anti–C1-INH autoantibodies. J Clin Invest 1989;83(6):1794–9.

[16] Cicardi M, Beretta A, Colombo M, et al. Relevance of lymphoproliferative disorders and of anti-C1 inhibitor autoantibodies in acquired angio-oedema. Clin Exp Immunol 1996;106(3): 475–80.

[17] Malbran A, Hammer CH, Frank MM, et al. Acquired angioedema: observations on the mechanism of action of autoantibodies directed against C1 esterase inhibitor. J Allergy Clin Immunol 1988;81(6):1199–204.

[18] Donaldson VH, Bernstein DI, Wagner CJ, et al. Angioneurotic edema with acquired C1- inhibitor deficiency and autoantibody to C1-inhibitor: response to plasmapheresis and cytotoxic therapy. J Lab Clin Med 1992;119(4):397–406.

[19] Zuraw BL, Curd JG. Demonstration of modified inactive first component of complement (C1) inhibitor in the plasmas of C1 inhibitor–deficient patients. J Clin Invest 1986;78(2): 567–75.

[20] Zuraw BL, Altman LC. Acute consumption of C1 inhibitor in a patient with acquired C1-inhibitor deficiency syndrome. J Allergy Clin Immunol 1991;88(6):908–18.

[21] Chatila TA. Role of regulatory T cells in human diseases. J Allergy Clin Immunol 2005; 116(5):949–59 [quiz: 960].

[22] Stone MJ, Merlini G, Pascual V. Autoantibody activity in Waldenstrom's macroglobuline-mia. Clin Lymphoma 2005;5(4):225–9.

[23] Smedby KE, Hjalgrim H, Askling J, et al. Autoimmune and chronic inflammatory disorders and risk of non-Hodgkin lymphoma by subtype. J Natl Cancer Inst 2006;98(1):51–60.

[24] Chevailler A, Arlaud G, Ponard D, et al. C1-inhibitor binding monoclonal immunoglobins in three patients with acquired angioneurotic edema. J Allergy Clin Immunol 1996;97(4): 998–1008.

[25] Hauptmann G, Lang JM, North ML, et al. Acquired C1-inhibitor deficiencies in lymphopro-liferative diseases with serum immunoglobulin abnormalities. A study of three cases. Blut 1976;32(3):195–206.

[26] Mathur R, Toghill PJ, Johnston ID. Acquired C1 inhibitor deficiency with lymphoma caus-ing recurrent angioedema. Postgrad Med J 1993;69(814):646–8.

[27] Bain BJ, Catovsky D, Ewan PW. Acquired angioedema as the presenting feature of lympho-proliferative disorders of mature B-lymphocytes. Cancer 1993;72(11):3318–22.

[28] Fremeaux-Bacchi V, Guinnepain MT, Cacoub P, et al. Prevalence of monoclonal gamm-opathy in patients presenting with acquired angioedema type 2. Am J Med 2002;113(3): 194–9.

[29] Monti G, Pioltelli P, Saccardo F, et al. Incidence and characteristics of non-Hodgkin lym-phomas in a multicenter case file of patients with hepatitis C virus–related symptomatic mixed cryoglobulinemias. Arch Intern Med 2005;165(1):101–5.

[30] Agostoni A, Cicardi M. Hereditary and acquired C1-inhibitor deficiency: biological and clin-ical characteristics in 235 patients. Medicine (Baltimore) 1992;71(4):206–15.

[31] Jackson J, Feighery C. Autoantibody-mediated acquired deficiency of C1 inhibitor. N Engl J Med 1988;318(2):122–3.

[32] Cohen SH, Koethe SM, Kozin F, et al. Acquired angioedema associated with rectal carci-noma and its response to danazol therapy. Acquired angioedema treated with danazol. J Al-lergy Clin Immunol 1978;62(4):217–21.

[33] Bouillet L, Ponard D, Drouet C, et al. [Acquired angioneurotic edema. Clinical and biolog-ical characteristics in 9 patients.]. Presse Med 2000;29(12):640–4 [in French].

[34] Dreyfus B, Kuentz M, Cordonnier C. [Apropos of the case reported by M. Leporrier et al., on mixed nodular lymphoma associated with a deficiency of C1-esterase inhibitor.] Nouv Rev Fr Hematol 1981;23(5):305–7 [in French].

[35] Gelfand JA, Boss GR, Conley CL, et al. Acquired C1 esterase inhibitor deficiency and an-gioedema: a review. Medicine (Baltimore) 1979;58(4):321–8.

[36] Nilsen A, Matre R. Acquired angioedema and hypocomplementemia in a patient with my-elofibrosis. Effect of danazol treatment. Acta Med Scand 1980;207(1–2):123–5.

[37] Schlaifer D, Arlet P, Montane de la Roque P, et al. Antiepileptic drug–induced lymphopro-liferative disorder associated with acquired C1 esterase inhibitor deficiency and angioedema. Eur J Haematol 1992;48(5):274–5.

[38] Sheffer AL, Austen KF, Rosen FS, et al. Acquired deficiency of the inhibitor of the first com-ponent of complement: report of five additional cases with commentary on the syndrome. J Allergy Clin Immunol 1985;75(6):640–6.

[39] Wasserfallen JB, Spaeth P, Guillou L, et al. Acquired deficiency in C1-inhibitor associated with signet ring cell gastric adenocarcinoma: a probable connection of antitumor-associated antibodies, hemolytic anemia, and complement turnover. J Allergy Clin Immunol 1995; 95(1 Pt 1):124–31.

[40] Cicardi M, Frangi D, Bergamaschini L, et al. Acquired C1 inhibitor deficiency with angioe-dema symptoms in a patient infected with Echinococcus granulosus. Complement 1985; 2(2–3):133–9.

[41] Casali P, Borzini P, Pioltelli P, et al. Acquired C1-inhibitor deficiency in essential cryoglobu-linemia and macrocryoglobulinemia. Acta Haematol 1978;59(5):277–84.

[42] Hauptmann G, Lang JM, North ML, et al. Lymphosarcoma, cold urticaria, IgG1 monoclo-nal cryoglobulin and complement abnormalities. Scand J Haematol 1975;15(1):22–6.

[43] Nagy L, Hannema A, Swaak A. Acquired C1 inhibitor deficiency associated with systemic lupus erythematosus, secondary antiphospholipid syndrome and IgM monoclonal paraproteinaemia. Clin Rheumatol 1999;18(1):56–8.

[44] Pascual M, Widmann JJ, Schifferli JA. Recurrent febrile panniculitis and hepatitis in two patients with acquired complement deficiency and paraproteinemia. Am J Med 1987;83(5): 959–62.

[45] Ordi-Ros J, Paredes J, Detarsio G, et al. Autoantibodies to C1 inhibitor in patients with lupus disease. J Rheumatol 1997;24(9):1856–8.

[46] Agostoni A, Aygoren-Pursun E, Binkley KE, et al. Hereditary and acquired angioedema: problems and progress: proceedings of the third C1 esterase inhibitor deficiency workshop and beyond. J Allergy Clin Immunol 2004;114(Suppl 3):S51–131.

[47] Cicardi M, Bisiani G, Cugno M, et al. Autoimmune C1 inhibitor deficiency: report of eight patients. Am J Med 1993;95(2):169–75.

[48] Gelfand JA, Sherins RJ, Alling DW, et al. Treatment of hereditary angioedema with danazol. Reversal of clinical and biochemical abnormalities. N Engl J Med 1976;295(26): 1444–8.

[49] Frank MM, Sergent JS, Kane MA, et al. Epsilon aminocaproic acid therapy of hereditary angioneurotic edema. A double-blind study. N Engl J Med 1972;286(15):808–12.

[50] Sheffer AL, Austen KF, Rosen FS. Tranexamic acid therapy in hereditary angioneurotic edema. N Engl J Med 1972;287(9):452–4.

[51] Cugno M, Cicardi M, Bottasso B, et al. Activation of the coagulation cascade in C1-inhibitor deficiencies. Blood 1997;89(9):3213–8.

[52] Cicardi M, Bergamaschini L, Zingale LC, et al. Idiopathic nonhistaminergic angioedema. Am J Med 1999;106(6):650–4.

[53] Bork K, Witzke G. Long-term prophylaxis with C1-inhibitor (C1 INH) concentrate in patients with recurrent angioedema caused by hereditary and acquired C1-inhibitor deficiency. J Allergy Clin Immunol 1989;83(3):677–82.

[54] Markovic SN, Inwards DJ, Frigas EA, et al. Acquired C1 esterase inhibitor deficiency. Ann Intern Med 2000;132(2):144–50.

[55] Bowen T, Cicardi M, Farkas H, et al. Canadian 2003 International Consensus Algorithm For the Diagnosis, Therapy, and Management of Hereditary Angioedema. J Allergy Clin Immunol 2004;114(3):629–37.

[56] Bork K, Barnstedt SE. Treatment of 193 episodes of laryngeal edema with C1 inhibitor concentrate in patients with hereditary angioedema. Arch Intern Med 2001;161(5): 714–8.

[57] Kunschak M, Engl W, Maritsch F, et al. A randomized, controlled trial to study the efficacy and safety of C1 inhibitor concentrate in treating hereditary angioedema. Transfusion 1998; 38(6):540–9.

[58] Waytes AT, Rosen FS, Frank MM. Treatment of hereditary angioedema with a vapor-heated C1 inhibitor concentrate. N Engl J Med 1996;334(25):1630–4.

[59] Han ED, MacFarlane RC, Mulligan AN, et al. Increased vascular permeability in C1 inhibitor–deficient mice mediated by the bradykinin type 2 receptor. J Clin Invest 2002;109(8): 1057–63.

[60] Shahar A, Sharon R, Lorber M, et al. [Angioedema caused by splenectomy with malignant lymphoma followed by multiple myeloma 7 years later.] Harefuah 1997;132(9) 624–626, 679 [in Hebrew].

[61] Postlethwaite KR, Parry DH. Acquired angioedema. Br J Oral Maxillofac Surg 1988;26(6): 499–502.

[62] Gottlieb M, Campbell K, Pelzmann K, et al. Long-standing angioedema with C1 esterase inhibitor deficiency associated with occult lymphoma. West J Med 1983;138(2): 258–60.

[63] van Spronsen DJ, Hoorntje SJ, Hannema AJ, et al. Acquired angio-oedema caused by IgA paraprotein. Neth J Med 1998;52(1):22–5.

[64] Boyar A, Zuraw BL, Beall G. Immunoadsorption in acquired angioedema: a therapeutic misadventure. Clin Immunol Immunopathol 1993;66(2):181–3.

[65] Frigas E. Angioedema with acquired deficiency of the C1 inhibitor: a constellation of syndromes. Mayo Clin Proc 1989;64(10):1269–75.

[66] Hentges F, Humbel R, Dicato M, et al. Acquired C1 esterase–inhibitor deficiency: case report with emphasis on complement and kallikrein activation during two patterns of clinical manifestations. J Allergy Clin Immunol 1986;78(5 Pt 1):860–7.

[67] Lipscombe TK, Orton DI, Bird AG, et al. Acquired C1-esterase inhibitor deficiency: three case reports and commentary on the syndrome. Australas J Dermatol 1996;37(3):145–8.

[68] Malcolm A, Prather CM. Intestinal angioedema mimicking Crohn's disease. Med J Aust 1999;171(8):418–20.

[69] Sinclair D, Smith A, Cranfield T, et al. Acquired C1 esterase inhibitor deficiency or serendipity? The chance finding of a paraprotein after an apparently low C1 esterase inhibitor concentration. J Clin Pathol 2004;57(4):445–7.

[70] Kleiner GI, Giclas P, Stadtmauer G, et al. Unmasking of acquired autoimmune C1-inhibitor deficiency by an angiotensin-converting enzyme inhibitor. Ann Allergy Asthma Immunol 2001;86(4):461–4.

[71] Spath PJ, Wuthrich B, Matter L, et al. Acquired angioedema and anti–C1-inhibitor autoantibody. Arch Intern Med 1989;149(5):1213–6.

[72] Valsecchi R, Reseghetti A, Pansera B, et al. Autoimmune C1 inhibitor deficiency and angioedema. Dermatology 1997;195(2):169–72.

[73] Delmer A, Garban F, Le Tourneau A, et al. Waldenstrom's macroglobulinemia with prominent splenomegaly and multiple immune disorders. Haematologica 1993;78(6):408–10.

[74] Rodriguez M, Ancochea J, De Buen C, et al. Acquired C1-inhibitor deficiency associated with a lupus-like anticoagulant activity. Ann Allergy 1988;61(5):348–50.

[75] Baldwin J, Pence HL, Karibo JM, et al. C1 esterase inhibitor deficiency: three presentations. Ann Allergy 1991;67(2 Pt 1):107–13.

[76] Hauptmann G, Mayer S, Lang JM, et al. Treatment of acquired C1-inhibitor deficiency with danazol. Ann Intern Med 1977;87(5):577–8.

[77] Rosenfeld SISP, Leddy JP. Angioedema and hypocomplementemia: unusual features of lymphoma. J Allergy Clin Immunol 1975;55:104.

[78] Richardson SG, Clarke CW, Gasson GB. Lymphocytic lymphoma and acquired C1 esterase inhibitor deficiency. Br J Dermatol 1989;120(1):121–4.

[79] Fiechtner JJ, Marx JJ Jr, Wolski KP, et al. Acquired angioedema, autoimmune hemolytic anemia, and lymphoma: resolution after therapy. Clin Immunol Immunopathol 1980; 15(4):642–5.

[80] Bohle W, Ruther U, Bokemeyer C, et al. Acquired C1–inhibitor deficiency with angioedema due to pleomorphic immunocytoma in a patient with three malignant tumors: long-term follow-up data and presentation of an additional case. Ann Hematol 1996;72(6):383–6.

[81] Gordon EH, Beall GN, Klaustermeyer WB. Angioedema and multiple myeloma. II. Ann Allergy 1983;51(3):378–80.

[82] Chevrant-Breton J, Mazeas D, Bagot M, et al. [Acquired angioneurotic edema caused by acquired deficiency of C1 esterase inhibitor disclosing lymphoproliferative syndrome. Apropos of a case, review of the literature.]. Ann Dermatol Venereol 1982;109(12):1049–56 [in French].

[83] Day NK, Winfield JB, Gee T, et al. Evidence for immune complexes involving anti-lymphocyte antibodies associated with hypocomplementaemia in chronic lymphocytic leukaemia (CLL). Clin Exp Immunol 1976;26(2):189–95.

[84] Gaur S, Cooley J, Aish L, et al. Lymphoma-associated paraneoplastic angioedema with normal C1-inhibitor activity: does danazol work? Am J Hematol 2004;77(3):296–8.

[85] Beretta KR, Spath PJ, Pedrazzini A, et al. [Angioedema due to acquired complement-C1-inhibitor deficiency in a female patient with non-Hodgkin lymphoma and autoimmune hemolytic anemia.]. Schweiz Med Wochenschr 1991;121(25):943–7 [in German].

[86] Lafeuillade A, Pellegrino P, Quilichini R. [Angioneurotic edema acquired during chronic lymphoid leukemia. A case.] Presse Med 1993;22(30):1421 [in French].

[87] Ochonisky S, Intrator L, Wechsler J, et al. Acquired C1 inhibitor deficiency revealing systemic lupus erythematosus. Dermatology 1993;186(4):261–3.

[88] Farkas H, Gyeney L, Majthenyi P, et al. Angioedema due to acquired C1-esterase inhibitor deficiency in a patient with Helicobacter pylori infection. Z Gastroenterol 1999;37(6):513–8.

[89] Ponce IM, Caballero T, Reche M, et al. Polyclonal autoantibodies against C1 inhibitor in a case of acquired angioedema. Ann Allergy Asthma Immunol 2002;88(6):632–7.

[90] Higa S, Hirata H, Minami S, et al. Autoimmune acquired form of angioedema that responded to danazol therapy. Intern Med 2002;41(5):398–402.

[91] Alonso JM, Fas MJ. Malignant bladder tumor transurethral resection in a patient with acquired C1 inhibitor deficiency. Acta Anaesthesiol Scand 2002;46(6):740–3.

[92] Cacoub P, Fremeaux-Bacchi V, De Lacroix I, et al. A new type of acquired C1 inhibitor deficiency associated with systemic lupus erythematosus. Arthritis Rheum 2001;44(8):1836–40.

[93] Szeplaki G, Varga L, Osvath L, et al. Deep venous thrombosis associated with acquired angioedema type II in a patient heterozygous for the mutation of factor V Leiden: effective treatment and follow-up for four years. Thromb Haemost 2006;95(5):898–9.

[94] Wautier JL, Ollier-Hartmann MP, Kadeva H, et al. First component of complement and thrombosis. Thromb Haemost 1981;45(3):247–51.

[95] Levi M, Hack CE, van Oers MH. Rituximab-induced elimination of acquired angioedema due to C1-inhibitor deficiency. Am J Med 2006;119(8):e3–5.

[96] Chadenat ML, Morelon S, Dupont C, et al. [Acquired angioneurotic edema: association with hydatidosis.] Presse Med 2000;29(16):1465 [in French].

ELSEVIER
SAUNDERS

Immunol Allergy Clin N Am
26 (2006) 691–708

IMMUNOLOGY
AND ALLERGY
CLINICS
OF NORTH AMERICA

Novel Therapies for Hereditary Angioedema

Bruce L. Zuraw, MD

*University of California San Diego, 9500 Gilman Drive, Mailcode 0732,
La Jolla, CA 92093-0732, USA*

Despite remarkable progress in understanding the molecular basis of C1 inhibitor (C1INH) deficiency (see article by Wagenaar-Bos and Hack elsewhere in this issue) and the mechanism of swelling in hereditary angioedema (HAE) (see article by Davis elsewhere in this issue), the pharmacologic options available for the treatment of HAE in the United States have remained virtually unchanged over the past 40 years [1,2]. Prophylactic use of alpha-alkylated androgens or anti-fibrinolytic agents are generally successful in decreasing the number and severity of angioedema attacks; however, these medications are associated with significant adverse effects and do not successfully address the treatment of acute attacks. Taken together, these problems indicate a significant unmet need for improved treatment options of HAE in the United States.

Fortunately, a variety of novel therapies for HAE are currently undergoing clinical evaluation for use in HAE under Food and Drug Administration (FDA) orphan drug designation. The rationale for the development and use of each of these novel molecules is based on the understanding of the molecular mechanisms that underlie HAE, suggesting that they will be more effective and safer then currently available treatments. This article will review the status of these emerging therapies, and provide a framework for considering their use in patients with HAE. These molecules define two separate approaches to the treatment of HAE: replacing the missing C1INH function; or inhibiting the kinin pathway that is responsible for the increased vascular permeability responsible for angioedema. Table 1 summarizes the key benefits and drawbacks of each of the molecules undergoing clinical trial for use in HAE.

This work was supported in part by Grants AI36220 and RR00833 from the National Institutes of Health.

E-mail address: bzuraw@ucsd.edu

0889-8561/06/$ - see front matter © 2006 Elsevier Inc. All rights reserved.
doi:10.1016/j.iac.2006.09.007

Table 1
Comparison of advantages and disadvantages of new drugs

Drug	Advantages	Disadvantages
Plasma-derived C1INH	Gold standard; extensive clinical experience; inhibits classical complement pathway and plasmin as well as bradykinin generation; long plasma half-life	Intravenous administration; potential viral/infectious contamination
rhC1INH	Same inhibitory spectrum as plasma-derived C1INH; no human viral/infectious risk; ability to be scaled up to easily produce as much product as needed	Intravenous administration; short half-life; risk of allergic reaction to contaminating rabbit protein; potential for xenotransmission of infectious agent
DX-88	More potent plasma kallikrein inhibitor than C1INH; no infectious risk; subcutaneous administration	May be antigenic; risk of anaphylactic reactions or development of neutralizing antibodies; short half-life; occasional nonresponder or rebound attack
Icatibant	Small peptide that is nonimmunogenic; no infectious risk; subcutaneous administration	Local discomfort at site of injection; short half-life; occasional nonresponder or rebound attack

Abbreviations: C1INH, C1 inhibitor; rh, recombinant human.

Replacement of C1 inhibitor

Rationale

In 1963, Donaldson and Evans demonstrated that the pathophysiologic basis of HAE was a deficiency of C1INH [3], a discovery that was soon recognized to also explain the lack of kallikrein inhibitory activity in HAE patient plasma observed the year before by Landerman et al [4]. While the precise mediator of the swelling remained an issue of some controversy for many years, it became immediately apparent that even partial replacement therapy to increase plasma C1INH levels could be an effective strategy to treat attacks of HAE. Early studies by Spath et al [5] demonstrated that plasma C1INH levels below 38% of normal were associated with evidence of enhanced complement activation. Anabolic androgens provided significant protection against attacks of angioedema when used at levels that increased plasma C1INH activity only marginally [6], thus suggesting that it was not necessary to normalize C1INH levels to achieve a good response. The success achieved by treatment of acute attacks of HAE with fresh frozen plasma (FFP) was also a harbinger of the potential efficacy of C1INH replacement therapy [7]. The clinical use of FFP, however, is complicated by questions regarding its safety with respect to viral or other infectious risk as well as concern by some investigators that under certain circumstances it can lead to rapid worsening of the angioedema. Taken together, these observations strongly supported the concept that C1INH replacement therapy can be used to treat attacks of angioedema.

While the major mediator of hereditary angioedema is almost certainly bradykinin (see article by Davis elsewhere in this issue), some investigators believe that other mediators may contribute to the vascular permeability defect. The efficacy of anti-fibronolytic drugs in prophylaxis has suggested to some that plasmin may also be important in triggering attacks. A theoretic advantage of C1INH therapy for acute attacks HAE compared with therapy directed against bradykinin generation or action is thus the ability of C1INH to inhibit complement proteases and plasmin in addition to contact system proteases.

Existing clinical experience with C1 inhibitor replacement therapy

Efficacy of plasma-derived C1 inhibitor

The efficacy of plasma C1INH as replacement therapy for acute attacks of HAE was confirmed more than 25 years ago [8–10]. Multiple other studies over the past 25 years have led to C1INH concentrates becoming the preferred modality of treatment for acute attacks of HAE in countries where it is available [11–14]. C1INH infusion results in an immediate increase in C1INH plasma levels, rapid improvement in symptoms (typically within 30 to 60 minutes), and a delayed increase in C4 levels (reflecting that this represents newly synthesized C4) [15–17]. The efficacy of C1INH concentrates appears to be equal for all types of HAE attacks, including laryngeal attacks where it can be lifesaving. Noteworthy in this regard is a report detailing the use of C1INH concentrate (Behrinert-P, ZLB Behring) for the treatment of 193 episodes of laryngeal angioedema in HAE patients without a single failure [12]. A history of 517 attacks of laryngeal angioedema was obtained in 42 patients from a cohort of 95 HAE patients. Of these, 193 episodes in 18 patients were treated with C1INH (500 to 1000 plasma units; 1 plasma unit is defined as being equal to the amount of C1INH in 1 mL of normal human plasma or approximately 270 µg/mL). Beginning of improvement in the laryngeal angioedema was noted in an average of 42.2 ± 19.9 minutes in the C1INH treated patients, and none of the treated patients required intubation. Resolution of the swelling symptoms occurred in an average of 15.3 ± 9.3 hours in the C1INH treated group compared with 100.8 ± 26.2 in the historical control group not treated with C1INH. Cicardi and Zingale [18] reported that C1INH concentrates were successful in the treatment for 629 of 630 acute attacks in their HAE population. They also point out that a beneficial response to C1INH infusion can be used as a reliable marker for the decision to avoid surgery and other expensive or invasive testing in patients with HAE who present with signs and symptoms of a possible "surgical abdomen."

Bork and colleagues [19] have also published a retrospective analysis of 131,110 angioedema attacks in 221 patients with HAE. Interestingly, the etiology of unusual symptoms (headache, urinary or renal retention/pain, muscle and joint swelling/pain, chest tightness/pressure, and painful swallowing) in this cohort was suggested to be angioedema by the ability of C1INH infusions to induce resolution of symptoms [19].

Four placebo-controlled double blind studies of C1INH for acute attacks of HAE have been performed. In 1996, Waytes and colleagues [20] published the results of two double-blind placebo-controlled studies comparing plasma-derived C1INH (25 plasma units/kg; Immuno AG) to placebo. The first was a crossover study involving prophylactic treatment of six severely affected HAE patients who received study drug every 3 days. Subjects were admitted for 17 days on two occasions (separated by at least 3 weeks), receiving five treatments during each admission. During the admission where they received C1INH, subjects increased their plasma C1INH functional levels, normalized their C4 titers, and had significantly less swelling than they did during the admission where they received placebo. The second study assessed the time to improvement following study drug in 22 patients with acute attacks of HAE. The beginning of relief occurred significantly faster in C1INH treated patients than in placebo-treated patients (55 versus 563 minutes). A third placebo-controlled randomized trial of Immuno C1INH by Kunschak and colleagues [17] also demonstrated efficacy of the C1INH compared with placebo in acute HAE attacks. Pharmacokinetic analysis of the Immuno C1INH in this study revealed an apparent half-life of 37.87 ± 19.75 hours during HAE attacks. Finally, a pivotal phase III trial of this drug, conducted by Baxter Health Care, surprisingly failed to show any improvement of the C1INH compared with placebo in acute HAE attacks. The failure of this study has been generally attributed to problems in the study design (60-minute crossover). Subsequent to this study, the Baxter C1INH product (identical to the Immuno C1INH) was withdrawn from the market worldwide.

Although C1INH is not available in the United States, current practice in Europe and Canada is to treat significant acute attacks of HAE with 500 to 1000 plasma units of C1INH by intravenous infusion [21]. The median functional half-life of infused C1INH has been estimated to be 4.48 days in healthy subjects, 46.5 hours in subjects with mild HAE, and 31.75 hours in subjects with severe HAE [21]. While not available as a licensed drug in the United States, a number of US patients import C1INH (Behrinert-P or Cetor) under the FDA personal importation program [22].

In addition to its use for acute attacks of HAE, C1 inhibitor concentrates have also been successfully used for both short-term and long-term prophylactic treatment of HAE. Long-term prophylaxis with C1INH may be particularly useful for patients with very severe disease and possibly during pregnancy in women who experience an increased frequency of attacks. Bork and Witzke [23] reported the successful use of C1INH concentrate for long-term prophylaxis in a patient with HAE with frequent attacks that could not be well controlled with androgens or anti-fibrinolytic drugs. Subsequently, other investigators have reported the successful use of long-term prophylactic C1INH (two to three times per week) for patients with severe HAE [21]. Long-term prophylaxis with C1INH has also been successfully used in pregnancy [24]. For short-term prophylaxis, purified C1INH should be at least as effective as fresh frozen plasma but with improved safety parameters. A number of reports have also demonstrated the efficacy of short-term prophylaxis with C1INH before dental work or surgery [25–28].

C1INH infusions have also been shown to be effective in the treatment of acute attacks of angioedema in patients with acquired C1INH deficiency. Even patients with acquired C1INH deficiency and anti-C1INH autoantibodies respond to C1INH infusion, although the dose may need to be increased in this setting [29]. As expected, however, C1INH infusion was shown to be ineffective in patients with type III HAE [30].

Because C1INH replacement requires intravenous administration of the drug, patients have needed to go to emergency rooms or physicians' offices to get the infusions. Because of the delay and inconvenience inherent in this approach to treatment, a number of investigators have allowed patients to self-administer C1INH at home after receiving instruction in proper technique. Self-administration of C1INH concentrate in patients with frequent or severe attacks of the angioedema for on-demand treatment of severe attacks (31 subjects, including 28 patients with HAE and 3 patients with acquired C1INH deficiency) or for prophylaxis (12 subjects, including 10 patients with HAE and 2 patients with acquired C1INH deficiency) was recently reported by Levi and colleagues [31]. Self-administration of C1INH was shown to be both effective and safe for both therapeutic and prophylactic use. Furthermore, the interval between onset of symptoms and initiation of therapy was significantly decreased in patients receiving self-administration (1.4 ± 1.0 hours) compared with conventional treatment (3.4 ± 2.1 hours). The earlier initiation of therapy was associated with a markedly reduced time to complete resolution of symptoms in patients during self-administration (5.9 ± 2.2 hours) compared with conventional treatment (13.8 ± 2.9 hours).

Safety of plasma-derived C1 inhibitor

C1INH concentrates are typically prepared from human plasma (except for the new recombinant transgenic C1INH; see the section "Recombinant transgenic human C1INH"); therefore, viral safety is a critical and ongoing issue that must be addressed prospectively and then continuously monitored. Before the incorporation of viral inactivation steps into the manufacturing process, cases of hepatitis C virus (HCV) transmission from C1INH concentrates were reported; however, this problem has been successfully addressed in the current group of concentrates by combining careful screening of plasma donors, a variety of viral inactivation steps during manufacturing, and polymerase chain reaction (PCR) monitoring for viral contamination. Cicardi and Zingale [18] report that more than 80% of patients receiving the earliest C1INH concentrates became infected with HCV (without any instance of documented HIV infection). In contrast, they report that use of a steam-heated C1INH (Immuno) in several hundred patients resulted in only a single case in which HCV conversion could not be excluded as being due to the concentrate. Waytes and colleagues [20] found no instances of seroconversion after 106 infusions of steam-heated C1INH (Immuno). A review of the use of pasteurized C1INH (Berinert P) between 1985 and 2003 found no documented cases of viral transmission [21].

Rare instances of anaphylactoid reactions to C1INH infusions have been reported [32]. Waytes and colleagues [20] screened for evidence of autoantibodies to C1 inhibitor that could have resulted from exposure to the concentrates in sera from all patients in their prophylaxis study and 13 patients in their treatment study. Notably, all samples were negative for anti-C1INH autoantibodies. Recently, elevated levels of IgM anti-C1INH autoantibodies were reported in patients with HAE compared with healthy controls; however, the titer of antibody did not bear any relationship to history of exposure to C1INH infusions [33].

Drugs in current clinical trials

Based on the demonstrated efficacy of C1INH concentrate therapy in HAE (virtually 100% response) together with the excellent safety profile of concentrates made using the newer manufacturing methods, licensing of C1INH replacement therapy in the United States is anticipated following a successful phase III study. There are three studies currently under way in the United States with the intent of leading to licensure of C1INH products. Each of these studies is briefly described below.

Plasma-derived C1 inhibitor concentrates

Lev Pharmaceuticals is conducting a phase III study of a nanofiltered pasteurized C1INH concentrate (C1INH-nf). This product is manufactured using a similar process as the current Cetor C1INH product (Sanguin). Cetor C1INH is widely used in The Netherlands, and has been shown to be extremely safe. The only difference between the C1INH-nf and Cetor products is the addition of a double nanofiltration step at the end of the purification for the C1INH-nf. Nanofiltration provides an extra margin of safety by excluding viral particles based on size rather than a particular physicochemical property of the virus. Nanofiltration is a robust and reliable viral reduction technique that predictably removes more than 4 to 6 logs of a wide range of viruses, including both enveloped and nonenveloped viruses [34]. There is also some data indicating that nanofiltration may remove prions [34]. The Lev C1 inhibitor in hereditary angioedema nanofiltration generation evaluating efficacy (CHANGE) study is composed of two separate randomized double-blind placebo-controlled studies of C1INH-nf.

The first is studying the efficacy and safety of C1INH-nf for the treatment of acute attacks of HAE. The second is a study of the efficacy of C1INH-nf for long-term prophylactic treatment of severe HAE.

ZLB Behring is conducting a phase II/III study of Behrinert P for the treatment of acute attacks of HAE. As reviewed above, Behrinert P has a long track record of safety and efficacy. The current study is a placebo-controlled, dose-finding, 3-arm, double-blind clinical trial in subjects with HAE during acute episodes of angioedema. The three treatment groups will receive one of the following: Behrinert P 10 U/kg, Behrinert P 20 U/kg, or placebo.

Recombinant transgenic human C1 inhibitor

Pharming Technologies BV (Leiden, The Netherlands) engineered rabbits that express a human C1INH transgene under the control of a mammary gland–specific promoter. The resulting transgenic recombinant human C1INH protein (rhC1INH) is secreted into the breast milk of female rabbits. Purification of the rhC1INH from the breast milk yields large amounts of human C1INH, which is fully functional but exhibits subtle differences in posttranslational glycosylation compared with plasma-derived human C1INH [35]. The rhC1INH was administered to 12 asymptomatic patients with HAE at doses ranging from 6.25 to 100 U/kg [36]. No side effects were observed, and the intravenous administration of this drug was associated with a rapid increase in functional plasma C1INH activity and a corresponding fall in C4 activation, followed by a slower increase in C4 levels. The half-life of the protein was dose dependent and was longest at the highest dose used (100 U/kg) where it was estimated to be 3 hours. The significantly faster clearance of rhC1INH from the plasma space compared with plasma-derived C1INH is presumably caused by the glycosylation differences in the transgenic protein.

A number of HAE patients have now been successfully treated for acute attacks of angioedema with the rhC1INH in an open-label phase II study, and a report of two successfully treated patients has been published [37]. Because the rhC1INH is purified from rabbit milk, there is potential concern regarding contamination of the C1INH concentrate with trace amounts of rabbit protein that could cause allergic reactions. The efficient purification process used by Pharming is suggested to minimize this risk, and a final assessment awaits further clinical experience. Based on the promising safety and efficacy data from the phase I and II studies, Pharming has now initiated a phase II/III study of its rhC1INH in the United States.

The potential advantages of rhC1INH include the ability to scale up production as needed and the freedom from potential contamination with viruses from human plasma. Whether the shorter plasma half-life of the rhC1INH has any clinical implications for treatment of acute attacks remains to be clearly demonstrated; however, the half-life of the rhC1INH would likely make this product less desirable than plasma-derived C1INH for prophylactic treatment.

Therapeutic uses of C1 inhibitor for conditions other than angioedema

C1INH is a broadly anti-inflammatory molecule [38], and it will likely be evaluated for its therapeutic potential in a variety of other situations. While the use of C1INH concentrates for nonangioedema indications is beyond the scope of this article, it has been reviewed in several recent articles [13,38–44].

Inhibition of bradykinin-mediated enhanced vascular permeability

Rationale

C1INH inhibits a number of different proteases, including the classical complement proteases C1r and C1s, the contact system proteases plasma kallikrein and factor XIIa (activated Hageman factor), the fibrinolytic protease plasmin, the coagulation factor X1a, and mannan-binding lectin (MBL)-associated serine proteases (MASPs). Most importantly, C1INH is the primary inhibitor of the complement proteases C1r and C1s and the contact system proteases plasma kallikrein and factor XIIa. During attacks of angioedema, a variety of abnormalities are seen in these proteolytic pathways. Activation of the early components of the classic complement pathway is a hallmark of HAE, and this is increased during episodes of angioedema. Similarly, contact system activation is seen during attacks of angioedema [45,46].

The mediator of angioedema in HAE was controversial for many years, with investigators favoring either C2-kinin (a product of complement plus plasmin activation) [47,48] or bradykinin (a product of contact system activation) [4,45,46,49–51]. As discussed in the article by Davis elsewhere in this issue, there is now very strong evidence that bradykinin is the major if not sole mediator of swelling in HAE. Based on the emerging consensus that bradykinin causes the swelling of HAE, therapeutic strategies to inhibit bradykinin generation or bradykinin action have been considered. Fig. 1 shows a schematic of the plasma contact system and demonstrates potential therapeutic modalities that may be useful to decrease bradykinin-mediated increases of vascular permeability. The first, C1INH replacement, has been reviewed above. The others, inhibition of plasma kallikrein activity and antagonism of the effect of bradykinin at its receptor, are reviewed below. The apparent efficacy of both of these drugs in treating acute attacks of HAE (see the following sections) strongly supports the previous scientific presumptions that bradykinin is the key mediator of angioedema in this disease.

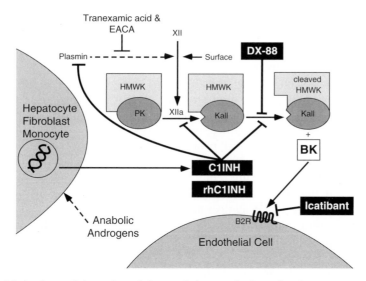

Fig. 1. Mechanisms of the action of the novel therapeutic drugs for the treatment of HAE based on their impact on bradykinin generation and effect. Plasma prekallikrein (PK) circulates in complex with high-molecular-weight kininogen (HMWK). Upon activation of the contact system, coagulation factor XII and prekallikrein are proteolytically activated to XIIa and kallikrein (Kall), respectively. Kallikrein then cleaves high-molecular-weight kininogen, releasing bradykinin (BK), the major active peptide involved in attacks. Bradykinin binds to bradykinin type 2 receptors (B2R) on endothelial cells, thereby increasing vascular permeability, which causes the edema. Anabolic androgens increase plasma levels of normal C1INH, although it is unclear whether this actually involves increased gene expression. Plasmin has been reported to release BK from HK, and the antifibrinolytics (EACA and tranexamic acid) may act by inhibiting activation of factor XII by plasmin. C1INH and rhC1INH inhibit both XIIa and kallikrein (as well as C1r, C1s, and plasmin). DX-88 specifically inhibits kallikrein, and Icatibant blocks binding of bradykinin to B2R on endothelial cells.

Plasma kallikrein inhibition

As discussed in the preceding section and reviewed in the accompanying chapter by Dr. Davis, activation of plasma kallikrein and generation of bradykinin appear to be the major cause of the increased vascular permeability in HAE. Inhibition of plasma kallikrein, which generates bradykinin from high molecular weight kininogen substrate, is thus a logical strategy to treat attacks of HAE. The first plasma kallikrein inhibitor, other than C1INH, to be used for the treatment of HAE was aprotinin (Trasylol), a broad spectrum serpin that has more potent inhibitory activity against trypsin and plasmin than it does against kallikrein. Aprotinin is primarily used in cardiac surgery to prevent excessive blood loss and inflammation. While aprotinin was shown to be effective for the treatment of acute attacks of HAE [10,52], it is a bovine protein (derived from cow lung) and its administration has been associated with severe anaphylactic reactions, rarely on first exposure, but particularly on repeated exposure [53,54]. The use of aprotinin for

HAE, which is characterized by repeated episodes of angioedema, is thus obviously contraindicated.

More recently, Dyax Inc identified a highly potent and specific inhibitor of plasma kallikrein by screening a phage display library consisting of rationally designed variants of the first Kunitz domain of human lipoprotein-associated coagulation inhibitor (LACI, also known as tissue factor pathway inhibitor) [55]. The resulting molecule, DX-88 (ecallantide), is a 60–amino acid protein with a molecular weight of 7054 Daltons that is produced as a recombinant protein in the yeast, *Pichia pastoris.* DX-88 is a reversible and highly potent plasma kallikrein inhibitor (apparent Ki for human plasma kallikrein of 44 pM compared with 13 nM for C1INH) that has a rapid on-rate (k_{on} 2×10^6 m^{-1}s^{-1}) and a slow off-rate (k_{on} 2×10^5 m^{-1}s^{-1}). Unlike aprotinin, DX-88 is also a highly specific plasma kallikrein inhibitor with an apparent Ki of at least 10 nM for 10 other human serine proteases. In three separate phase I protocols, DX-88 was demonstrated to be well tolerated with consistent pharmacokinetics. At a dose of 20 mg given intravenously, DX-88 had a half-life of approximately 72 minutes. DX-88 was subsequently reformulated as a subcutaneous rather than an intravenous drug. As anticipated, the subcutaneous formulation showed a longer half-life (2 hours) than the intraveneous formulation.

The efficacy of DX-88 for the treatment of C1INH deficiency has been demonstrated in several different models. When given to C1INH null mice, DX-88 almost completely abrogated the chronic vascular permeability defect observed in these animals [56]. DX-88 has been studied in three different phase II protocols. The first (EDEMA0) was an open-label phase study involving nine HAE subjects in which intravenous DX-88 treatment resulted in improvement of symptoms in a time frame similar to that seen for C1INH concentrates. The second phase II study (EDEMA1) was a placebo-controlled randomized double-blind escalating single-dose protocol assessing the efficacy of ascending doses (5, 10, 20, and 40 mg/m^2) of intravenous DX-88 in 48 HAE subjects. This study confirmed that DX-88 had a statistically significant beneficial effect for the treatment of acute attacks of HAE. DX-88–treated subjects were significantly more likely to report improvement within 4 hours of dosing (72.5% responders; median time to improvement 70 minutes) than were placebo-treated subjects (25%; median time to improvement 246 minutes). The final phase II study (EDEMA2) was an open-label multiple treatment extension protocol. An interim analysis of EDEMA2 involving 180 attacks in 63 subjects demonstrated the following response rates: 92% at 5 mg/m^2 intravenously (IV) (n = 24), 86% at 10 mg/m^2 IV (n = 135), and 100% at 20 mg/m^2 IV (n = 15) and 30 mg subcutaneously (n = 6). Median time to improvement was 30 minutes. A phase III study (EDEMA3), using 30 mg of the subcutaneous DX-88 for the treatment of acute attacks of HAE, is currently ongoing in the United States.

DX-88 is also being studied in cardiac surgery where early data indicate that it is able to decrease blood loss. DX-88 has also recently shown beneficial activity in preventing cerebral ischemia-reperfusion injury in a murine model [57].

More than 450 doses of DX-88 have been successfully given to more than 180 HAE subjects, and the drug appears to be generally well tolerated. Nevertheless, a few concerns have arisen. Unlike C1INH, there appear to be rare attacks that may not respond to DX-88; and several subjects have experienced "rebound" angioedema, ie, a return of angioedema symptoms a number of hours after apparent response to the drug. Interestingly, the "rebound" angioedema appears to be primarily associated with lower doses of DX-88 and thus may not be a substantial issue as experience with the 30-mg subcutaneous dose increases.

Prolongation of the aPTT is commonly seen, representing a pharmacologic effect of the drug without any enhanced risk of bleeding. There have been eight reports of mild anaphylactic-like reactions to first-dose exposure to DX-88, and at least some of these may have been related to the speed of infusion. Tryptase levels following these reactions have been universally negative. Patients who experienced acute dosing reactions all showed improvement in their HAE symptoms, and several of them received subsequent treatment with DX-88 without adverse reaction of loss of efficacy. Two of the subjects who experienced acute dosing reactions were found by Dyax to have antibodies to the study drug: one had non-IgE antibodies to DX-88 and the other had anti-*Pichia pastoris* IgE antibodies. Both of these subjects underwent DX-88 rechallenge without problems. There is also one report of a first-dose anaphylactic-like reaction that was associated with serum antibodies to a low molecular component of the drug (IgE, IgG, IgM, and IgA) detected by immunoblotting [58]. Using a validated ELISA, Dyax was unable to confirm antibodies against either DX-88 or *P pastoris* in this subject [59], and studies are ongoing to resolve this issue. Eleven subjects have developed detectable anti-DX-88 antibodies, seven to contaminating *P pastoris* proteins, three to the DX-88 itself, and one to both. Two of the subjects with anti-DX-88 protein antibodies have continued to receive DX-88 open-label treatment without adverse effect or loss of efficacy. Furthermore, changes in the manufacturing process have been reported to have reduced the contamination with *P pastoris* proteins by 2 orders of magnitude.

Bradykinin receptor antagonist

DX-88 inhibits plasma kallikrein, the protease that cleaves high molecular weight kininogen (HMWK) and releases bradykinin. Blocking the biologic actions of bradykinin at the level of its receptor (the bradykinin B2 receptor) on endothelial cells represents an alternative therapeutic strategy. A variety of potent small bradykinin B2 receptor antagonists have been synthesized [60,61]. Icatibant (Hoe 140; d-Arg[Hyp3,Thi5, d-Tic7, Oic8]- bradykinin) is a synthetic decapeptide second-generation bradykinin B2 receptor antagonist that displays high affinity, little residual agonist activity, and an impressive resistance to peptidases (due to the use of non-natural amino acids in its backbone) [62]. Based on its demonstrated ability to antagonize bradykinin effects at the B2 receptor, the use of B2 receptor antagonists for the treatment of HAE has been under discussion for a number of years.

Treatment of C1INH null mice with Hoe-140 corrected the permeability defect seen in these animals [56]. Hoe-140, furthermore, has been safely administered to more than 700 human subjects for a variety of indications. Based on all of these considerations, Icatibant was identified by Jerini AG as a promising therapeutic drug for the treatment of HAE attacks.

An initial Phase I study of intravenous Icatibant showed that it was safe, highly bioavailable, and had excellent vascular distribution. Subsequently, Jerini developed a subcutaneous formulation of Icatibant that had similar safety and pharmacokinetic parameters. Interestingly, the subcutaneous formulation of Icatibant is stable at room temperature for at least 1 year.

Phase II studies performed in Europe by Jerini suggested that Icatibant was effective in abrogating acute angioedema attacks in eight patients with HAE. An initial open-label phase II study showed efficacy in eight attacks of HAE. A follow-up phase II study assessed the efficacy of five different doses of intravenous or subcutaneous Icatibant in patients with HAE experiencing attacks of angioedema (four subjects per group). Results of this study are expressed as the time to beginning of relief/time to complete resolution of symptoms, and were as follows: 0.4 mg/kg intravenously over 2 hours, 90 min/435 min; 0.4 mg/kg intravenously over 30 minutes, 85 min/1050 min; 0.8 mg/kg intravenously over 30 minutes, 67 min/833 min; 30 mg subcutaneously, 35 min/770 min; 45 mg subcutaneously, 27 min/1202 min. In contrast, the times to beginning of relief and time to complete resolution for historical matched untreated attacks were 34 hours and 3.25 days, respectively.

More than 300 subcutaneous open-label treatments with Icatibant have been administered for abdominal, cutaneous, and laryngeal HAE attacks. The vast majority of subjects treated with open-label Icatibant responded completely and did not require additional therapy. In one series, 9% of subjects receiving open-label drug required additional treatments. Interestingly, 20 subjects received open-label Icatibant for laryngeal angioedema, and all reported rapid relief with no need for re-treatment.

Jerini initiated two phase III studies (FAST-1 and FAST-2) for the treatment of acute HAE attacks using the subcutaneous formulation of Icatibant. One study compared Icatibant to placebo in the United States, Argentina, Australia, and Canada. The other study compared Icatibant to tranexamic acid in Europe and Israel. Preliminary analyses of the results revealed that subjects receiving Icatibant in the FAST-1 study reported improvement in a median time of 2.5 hours compared to 4.6 hours in placebo treated subjects ($p = 0.131$). In the FAST-2 study, subjects receiving

Icatibant experienced onset of relief in 2.0 hours compared to 12.0 hours in subjects receiving tranexemic acid ($p < 0.001$). Both studies are now continuing in an open-label extension phase. Icatibant is also being pursued as a potential therapeutic modality for a variety of inflammatory diseases including asthma, liver disease, and severe burns [63,64].

Icatibant has been tested in various formulations in a variety of diseases and has been shown to be safe and well tolerated in more than 1100 subjects to date. The current 30-mg subcutaneous dose has been administered in over 300 treatments, also with good tolerability, although some subjects complain of local pain and redness at the injection site. These local reactions are self-limited and have not required any specific treatment.

Future considerations regarding the treatment of hereditary angioedema

Current treatment options for patients with HAE are severely limited, and associated with significant side effects. Successful completion and licensing of some or all of the discussed drugs will provide new opportunities for treating patients with HAE that should help resolve this unmet need. To begin to address how HAE treatment might be optimally managed, several guidelines can be defined that may help in choosing the optimal treatment strategy. First, it is crucial that patients with HAE be treated in a manner that maximizes their health while minimizing potential side effects. Second, the treatment of HAE patients should be individualized. And third, treatment decisions should take into account the disruption of normal life caused by attacks of angioedema. Table 2 summarizes how these new drugs might be used to treat HAE.

Some of the implications of maximizing the health of patients with HAE while minimizing potential side effects are obvious. Thus, it is clear that effective therapy for severe or life-threatening attacks of angioedema must be readily available to patients with HAE. Similarly, use of high doses of anabolic androgens or anti-fibrinolytic drugs are predictably associated with potentially severe side effects, and thus should be avoided. Perhaps less obviously, it will also be crucial to improve the recognition and diagnosis of HAE among caregivers as many patients with HAE are believed to remain undiagnosed. In addition, the particular morbidity associated with the use of anabolic androgens in women raises the possibility that these drugs (that have been the main treatment modality for HAE) may become relatively contraindicated in women.

The likelihood of having multiple effective medications for the treatment of HAE offers the possibility of individualizing therapeutic strategy. Patients may require different therapeutic approaches based on a number of parameters, including differences in attack frequency or severity, differences in response to individual therapeutic agents due to pharmacogenetics, and differences in the ability of patients to tolerate acute attacks

Table 2
Utilization of new drugs

Scenario	Indication	Best drugs	Comment
Acute attack, treated at home	Preferred method of treating attacks to minimize interval between symptom onset and definitive treatment	DX-88 and Icatibant may be preferred because of ease of self-administration	There is strong precedent for patients/families learning to self-administer intravenously, which would allow plasma-derived C1INH and rhC1INH to also be ideal drugs for this use
Acute attack, treated in medical facility	Patients who present in medical facility with an attack either primarily or after failure of home therapy	Plasma-derived C1INH	C1INH replacement is likely to remain the gold standard treatment when one wants to definitively treat an attack without risk of rebound. If clinical studies show that rhC1INH is as effective as plasma-derived C1INH without nonresponders or rebound attacks, then this drug may become the preferred treatment in this scenario.
Short-term prophylaxis	Before extensive dental work, invasive procedures, or surgery	Plasma-derived C1INH	C1INH replacement has been shown to be effective in this situation. Additional experience with the other drugs may expand the recommended drug list.
Long-term prophylaxis	Patients with very severe or frequent attacks who cannot be controlled with or cannot tolerate low-dose anabolic androgens, especially pregnant patients, women, and children	Plasma-derived C1INH	C1INH replacement is likely to remain the only recommended treatment for long-term prophylaxis.

because of age, pregnancy, coexisting medical conditions, or access to medical care. Individualization of therapy will involve the specific medication used as well as the schedule of usage (for acute attacks versus prophylactic).

Finally, optimal treatment must attempt to limit the disruption of normal life that occurs in many patients with HAE. School or work absence is a major issue for patients, and preventing such absences is an important therapeutic goal. Since the natural history of HAE attacks evolves typically over approximately 3 days, many patients suffer substantial absences from school or work. Such absences are not confined to severe attacks, as HAE attacks involving the dominant hand or bottom of the feet can also make it impossible to work or go to school. In addition, there are compelling data suggesting that the time to complete resolution of angioedema symptoms is strongly influenced by the interval between onset of symptoms and institution of effective therapy [31]. Thus, the availability of self-administration (whether subcutaneously or intravenously) of an effective therapeutic agent early in an attack will likely be a key issue in optimal care of patients. Self-administration can obviate the need for patients to go to hospitals, emergency rooms, or even physician offices during an acute attack and thus dramatically shorten this important interval.

A significant fraction of patients with HAE in the United States are either not adequately controlled on currently available therapy or require doses of medications that expose them to the risk of serious side effects. All HAE patients, moreover, are at risk of having severe episodes of angioedema (potentially including life-threatening attacks involving their airway), for which there is currently no specific treatment available in the United States. Based on significant advances in understanding of HAE pathogenesis, novel therapies for HAE have been developed that promise much more specific and effective therapy than what has previously been available. The emergence of drugs that specifically address the pathophysiology of HAE thus has important implications for the management of these patients. Replacement therapy with purified plasma-derived or recombinant C1INH or treatment with a recombinant plasma kallikrein inhibitor or bradykinin B2 receptor antagonist each show the potential to provide reliable control of acute attacks of angioedema. In addition, C1INH replacement therapy provides new possibilities for both short-term and long-term prophylaxis. The availability of these new therapies could also obviate many of the most difficult problems encountered in treating patients with HAE, particularly for children and pregnant women. To take full advantage of these opportunities, however, clinicians and health care systems will need to radically change their existing algorithms for the care of HAE patients. Ultimately, the availability of these drugs coupled with patient-centric treatment plans should allow patients to reap the benefits of improved health with fewer side effects.

References

[1] Nilsson IM, Andersson L, Bjorkman SE. Epsilon-aminocaproic acid (E-ACA) as a therapeutic agent based on 5 years' clinical experience. Acta Med Scand Suppl 1966;448:1–46.

[2] Spaulding WB. Methyltestosterone therapy for hereditary episodic edema (hereditary angioneurotic edema). Ann Intern Med 1960;53:739–45.

[3] Donaldson VH, Evans RR. A biochemical abnormality in hereditary angioneurotic edema: absence of serum inhibitor of C'1- esterase. Am J Med 1963;35:37–44.

[4] Landerman NS, Webster ME, Becker EL, et al. Hereditary angioneurotic edema. II. Deficiency of inhibitor for serum globulin permeability factor and/or plasma kallikrein. J Allergy 1962;33:330–41.

[5] Spath PJ, Wuthrich B, Butler R. Quantification of C1-inhibitor functional activities by immunodiffusion assay in plasma of patients with hereditary angioedema—evidence of a functionally critical level of C1-inhibitor concentration. Complement 1984;1:147–59.

[6] Sheffer AL, Fearon DT, Austen KF. Hereditary angioedema: a decade of management with stanozolol. J Allergy Clin Immunol 1987;80:855–60.

[7] Pickering RJ, Good RA, Kelly JR, et al. Replacement therapy in hereditary angioedema. Successful treatment of two patients with fresh frozen plasma. Lancet 1969;1:326–30.

[8] Agostoni A, Bergamaschini L, Martignoni G, et al. Treatment of acute attacks of hereditary angioedema with C1-Inhibitor concentrate. Ann Allergy 1980;44:299–301.

[9] Gadek JE, Hosea SW, Gelfand JA, et al. Replacement therapy in hereditary angioedema. Successful treatment of acute episodes of angioedema with partly purified C1 inhibitor. N Engl J Med 1980;302:542–6.

[10] Marasini B, Cicardi M, Martignoni GC, et al. Treatment of hereditary angioedema. Klin Wochenschr 1978;56:819–23.

[11] Bergamaschini L, Cicardi M, Tucci A, et al. C1 INH concentrate in the therapy of hereditary angioedema. Allergy 1983;38:81–4.

[12] Bork K, Barnstedt SE. Treatment of 193 episodes of laryngeal edema with C1 inhibitor concentrate in patients with hereditary angioedema. Arch Intern Med 2001;161:714–8.

[13] Kirschfink M, Mollnes TE. C1-inhibitor: an anti-inflammatory reagent with therapeutic potential. Expert Opin Pharmacother 2001;2:1073–83.

[14] Logan RA, Greaves MW. Hereditary angio-oedema: treatment with C1 esterase inhibitor concentrate. J R Soc Med 1984;77:1046–8.

[15] Agostoni A, Cicardi M. Hereditary and acquired C1-inhibitor deficiency: biological and clinical characteristics in 235 patients. Medicine (Baltimore) 1992;71:206–15.

[16] Bork K, Hardt J, Schicketanz KH, et al. Clinical studies of sudden upper airway obstruction in patients with hereditary angioedema due to C1 esterase inhibitor deficiency. Arch Intern Med 2003;163:1229–35.

[17] Kunschak M, Engl W, Maritsch F, et al. A randomized, controlled trial to study the efficacy and safety of C1 inhibitor concentrate in treating hereditary angioedema. Transfusion 1998; 38:540–9.

[18] Cicardi M, Zingale L. How do we treat patients with hereditary angioedema? Transfus Apher Sci 2003;29:221–7.

[19] Bork K, Meng G, Staubach P, et al. Hereditary angioedema: new findings concerning symptoms, affected organs, and course. Am J Med 2006;119:267–74.

[20] Waytes AT, Rosen FS, Frank MM. Treatment of hereditary angioedema with a vapor-heated C1 inhibitor concentrate. N Engl J Med 1996;334:1630–4.

[21] De Serres J, Groner A, Lindner J. Safety and efficacy of pasteurized C1 inhibitor concentrate (Berinert P) in hereditary angioedema: a review.jean.de.serres@aventis.com. Transfus Apheresis Sci 2003;29:247–54.

[22] US HAE Association. C1-inhibitor (C1INH) personal importation. Available at: http://www.hereditaryangioedema.com/import.html. Accessed October 20, 2006.

[23] Bork K, Witzke G. Long-term prophylaxis with C1-inhibitor (C1 INH) concentrate in patients with recurrent angioedema caused by hereditary and acquired C1-inhibitor deficiency. J Allergy Clin Immunol 1989;83:677–82.

[24] Altman AD, McLaughlin J, Schellenberg R, et al. Hereditary angioedema managed with low-dose danazol and C1 esterase inhibitor concentrate: a case report. J Obstet Gynaecol Can 2006;28:27–31.

[25] Lehmann A, Lang J, Boldt J, et al. Successful off-pump coronary artery bypass graft surgery in a patient with hereditary angioedema. J Cardiothorac Vasc Anesth 2002; 16:473–6.

[26] Leimgruber A, Jaques WA, Spaeth PJ. Hereditary angioedema: uncomplicated maxillofacial surgery using short-term C1 inhibitor replacement therapy. Int Arch Allergy Immunol 1993; 101:107–12.

[27] Maves KK, Weiler JM. Tonsillectomy in a patient with hereditary angioedema after prophylaxis with C1 inhibitor concentrate. Ann Allergy 1994;73:435–8.

[28] Mohr M, Pollok-Kopp B, Gotze O, et al. [The use of a C1-inhibior concentrate for short-term preoperative prophylaxis in two patients with hereditary angioedema.]. Anaesthesist 1996;45:626–30 [in German].

[29] Alsenz J, Lambris JD, Bork K, et al. Acquired C1 inhibitor (C1-INH) deficiency type II. Replacement therapy with C1-INH and analysis of patients' C1-INH and anti-C1-INH autoantibodies. JCI 1989;83:1794–9.

[30] Bork K, Barnstedt SE, Koch P, et al. Hereditary angioedema with normal C1-inhibitor activity in women. Lancet 2000;356:213–7.

[31] Levi M, Choi G, Picavet C, et al. Self-administration of C1-inhibitor concentrate in patients with hereditary or acquired angioedema caused by C1-inhibitor deficiency. J Allergy Clin Immunol 2006;117:904–8.

[32] Bergamaschini L, Cicardi M. Recent advances in the use of C1 inhibitor as a therapeutic agent. Mol Immunol 2003;40:155–8.

[33] Varga L, Szeplaki G, Visy B, et al. C1-inhibitor (C1-INH) autoantibodies in hereditary angioedema Strong correlation with the severity of disease in C1-INH concentrate naive patients. Mol Immunol 2007;44:1454–60.

[34] Burnouf T, Radosevich M. Nanofiltration of plasma-derived biopharmaceutical products. Haemophilia 2003;9:24–37.

[35] Koles K, van Berkel PH, Pieper FR, et al. N- and O-glycans of recombinant human C1 inhibitor expressed in the milk of transgenic rabbits. Glycobiology 2004;14:51–64.

[36] van Doorn MB, Burggraaf J, van Dam T, et al. A phase I study of recombinant human C1 inhibitor in asymptomatic patients with hereditary angioedema. J Allergy Clin Immunol 2005;116:876–83.

[37] Porebski G, Bilo B, Obtulowicz K, et al. [Recombinant human C1-inhibitor is effective in the treatment of acute attacks of hereditary angioedema–case report]. Przegl Lek 2005;62: 317–20 [in Polish].

[38] Caliezi C, Wuillemin WA, Zeerleder S, et al. C1-Esterase inhibitor: an anti-inflammatory agent and its potential use in the treatment of diseases other than hereditary angioedema. Pharmacol Rev 2000;52:91–112.

[39] Cai S, Davis AE 3rd. Complement regulatory protein C1 inhibitor binds to selectins and interferes with endothelial-leukocyte adhesion. J Immunol 2003;171:4786–91.

[40] Cicardi M, Zingale L, Zanichelli A, et al. C1 inhibitor: molecular and clinical aspects. Springer Semin Immunopathol 2005;27:286–98.

[41] Horstick G. C1-esterase inhibitor in ischemia and reperfusion. Immunobiology 2002;205: 552–62.

[42] Kirschfink M. C1-inhibitor and transplantation. Immunobiology 2002;205:534–41.

[43] Liu D, Cai S, Gu X, et al. C1 inhibitor prevents endotoxin shock via a direct interaction with lipopolysaccharide. J Immunol 2003;171:2594–601.

[44] Storini C, Rossi E, Marrella V, et al. C1-inhibitor protects against brain ischemia-reperfusion injury via inhibition of cell recruitment and inflammation. Neurobiol Dis 2005;19:10–7.

[45] Schapira M, Silver LD, Scott CF, et al. Prekallikrein activation and high-molecular-weight kininogen consumption in hereditary angioedema. N Engl J Med 1983;308:1050–4.

[46] Zuraw BL, Curd JG. Demonstration of modified inactive first component of complement (C1) inhibitor in the plasmas of C1 inhibitor-deficient patients. JCI 1986;78:567–75.

[47] Donaldson VH, Ratnoff OD, Da Silva WD, et al. Permeability-increasing activity in hereditary angioneurotic edema plasma. II. Mechanism of formation and partial characterization. JCI 1969;48:642–53.

[48] Donaldson VH, Rosen FS, Bing DH. Role of the second component of complement (C2) and plasmin in kinin release in hereditary angioneurotic edema (H.A.N.E.) plasma. Trans Assoc Am Physicians 1977;40:174–83.

[49] Curd JG, Prograis LJ Jr, Cochrane CG. Detection of active kallikein in induced blister fluids of hereditary angioedema patients. J Exp Med 1980;152:742–7.

[50] Curd JG, Yelvington M, Burridge N, et al. Generation of bradykinin during incubation of hereditary angioedema plasma. Mol Immunol 1983;19:1365.

[51] Fields T, Ghebrehiwet B, Kaplan AP. Kinin formation in hereditary angioedema plasma: evidence against kinin derivation from C2 and in support of "spontaneous" formation of bradykinin. J Allergy Clin Immunol 1983;72:54–60.

[52] Juhlin L, Michaelsson G. Use of a kallikrein inhibitor in the treatment of urticaria and hereditary angioneurotic edema. Acta Derm Venereol 1969;49:37–44.

[53] Bauer J, Futterman S, Dreiling DA. Anaphylactic shock secondary to initial Trasylol administration. Am J Gastroenterol 1971;56:542–4.

[54] Proud G, Chamberlain J. Anaphylactic reaction to aprotinin [letter]. Lancet 1976;2:48–9.

[55] Williams A, Baird LG. DX-88 and HAE: a developmental perspective. Transfus Apheresis Sci 2003;29:255–8.

[56] Han ED, MacFarlane RC, Mulligan AN, et al. Increased vascular permeability in C1 inhibitor-deficient mice mediated by the bradykinin type 2 receptor. J Clin Invest 2002;109: 1057–63.

[57] Storini C, Bergamaschini L, Gesuete R, et al. Selective inhibition of plasma kallikrein protects brain from reperfusion injury. J Pharmacol Exp Ther 2006;318:849–54.

[58] Caballero T, Lopez-Serrano C. Anaphylactic reaction and antibodies to DX-88 (kallikrein inhibitor) in a patient with hereditary angioedema. J Allergy Clin Immunol 2006;117:476–7.

[59] Beck TR, Baird LG. Reply: anaphylactic reaction and antibodies to DX-88 (kallikrein inhibitor) in a patient with hereditary angioedema. J Allergy Clin Immunol 2006;117:477.

[60] Stewart JM, Gera L, Hanson W, et al. A new generation of bradykinin antagonists. Immunopharmacology 1996;33:51–60.

[61] Stewart JM, Vavrek RJ. Kinin antagonists: design and activities. J Cardiovasc Pharmacol 1990;15:S69–74.

[62] Hock FJ, Wirth K, Albus U, et al. Hoe 140 a new potent and long acting bradykinin-antagonist: in vitro studies. Br J Pharmacol 1991;102:769–73.

[63] Akbary AM, Wirth KJ, Schölkens BA. Efficacy and tolerability of Icatibant (Hoe 140) in patients with moderately severe chronic bronchial asthma. Immunopharmacology 1996;33: 238–42.

[64] Moreau ME, Garbacki N, Molinaro G, et al. The kallikrein-kinin system: current and future pharmacological targets. J Pharmacol Sci 2005;99:6–38.

ELSEVIER
SAUNDERS

Immunol Allergy Clin N Am
26 (2006) 709–724

IMMUNOLOGY
AND ALLERGY
CLINICS
OF NORTH AMERICA

Hereditary Angioedema with Normal C1 Inhibitor Activity Including Hereditary Angioedema with Coagulation Factor XII Gene Mutations

Konrad Bork, MD

*Department of Dermatology, Johannes Gutenberg University,
Langenbeckstr 1, 55131 Mainz, Germany*

Recurrent angioedema of the skin is a commonly diagnosed clinical symptom that can be found in various clinical entities [1,2]. Some types of angioedema of the skin are associated with episodes of upper airway obstruction that may be life threatening. Death by asphyxiation from laryngeal edema is well known in hereditary angioedema (HAE) due to C1 inhibitor deficiency [3,4] and in recurrent angioedema induced by angiotensin-converting enzyme (ACE) inhibitors [5–9]. Therefore, it is important to determine the exact type of angioedema in each patient.

In many patients angioedema is associated with urticaria. If relapsing urticaria occurs simultaneously or alternately with angioedema, both conditions are assumed to be symptoms of the same disease. This assumption is true in chronic idiopathic urticaria/angioedema, IgE-mediated reactions (to foods, drugs, insect toxins, and other substances), serum sickness, urticaria/angioedema induced by aspirin and nonsteroidal anti-inflammatory drugs (NSAIDS) or azo dyes and benzoates, and in reactions caused by substances that induce direct histamine release from mast cells.

Recurrent angioedema may occur in patients without urticaria. In these cases various disease entities due to a number of different pathogenetic mechanisms have to be considered. Recurrent angioedema without urticaria can be due to an inherited or acquired C1 inhibitor deficiency [10–13] or may be induced by ACE inhibitors. HAE due to C1 inhibitor deficiency is not associated with urticaria, whereas ACE inhibitors may cause recurrent angioedema alone or in association with urticaria. Other types of angioedema without urticaria

E-mail address: bork@hautklinik.klinik.uni-mainz.de

doi:10.1016/j.iac.2006.09.003   *immunology.theclinics.com*

include local angioedema secondary to physical stress such as vibratory angioedema. A group of patients remains with recurrent angioedema whose clinical symptoms cannot be ascribed to one of these disorders; this type of angioedema is referred to as "idiopathic angioedema" [2,14].

Until recently it was assumed that hereditary angioedema is a disease that results exclusively from a deficiency of the C1 inhibitor. In 1985, the author of this article observed a large family in which five women suffered from recurrent angioedema of the skin associated with relapsing episodes of abdominal pain attacks and episodes of upper airway obstruction. Surprisingly, all of the women had normal C1 inhibitor function. One of the family members had asphyxiated secondary to sudden laryngeal edema. Since then the author has paid special attention to similar patients. In 2000, 10 families with this disease were described [15]. In these families a total of 36 women, but not a single man, were affected. All patients had normal C1 inhibitor concentration and activity with respect to C1 esterase inhibition, ruling out both types of HAE (HAE type I and HAE type II). We proposed to call this hitherto unknown disease "hereditary angioedema with normal C1 inhibitor occurring mainly in women" or "hereditary angioedema type III." However, we were aware that this denomination (HAE type III) might be a generic diagnosis and might turn out to include various clinicogenetic entities. Subsequently, two additional families were described, with seven affected women in one family and four in the other [16,17]. Recently, clinical data on an additional 29 women with HAE type III were presented [18]. Because all 76 patients from the studies cited above were women, it was assumed that the clinical phenotype might be limited to the female sex. However, in 2006 we described a family with dominantly inherited angioedema and normal C1 inhibitor in which not only five female but also three male family members were clinically affected [19].

Our recent results of molecular genetics revealed mutations in the coagulation factor XII (Hageman factor) gene in the affected women in some families with "hereditary angioedema with normal C1 inhibitor" [20]. These patients have "hereditary angioedema with coagulation factor XII gene mutations" and represent a subgroup of "hereditary angioedema with normal C1 inhibitor." Other patients from additional families (see Genetic results) do not have these mutations; we assume a genetic heterogeneity in patients with "hereditary angioedema with normal C1 inhibitor" [20].

Clinical presentation

Clinical symptoms

The clinical symptoms include recurrent skin swellings (Fig. 1), abdominal pain attacks, tongue swellings, and laryngeal edema. Until now, only a relatively small number of patients and families have been described. In 2000, we reported that 36 patients exhibited relapsing skin swellings or

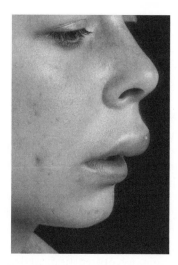

Fig. 1. Lip swelling in a patient with hereditary angioedema with normal C1 inhibitor (HAE type III). This was the third lip swelling during the 1-year-long intake of an oral contraceptive.

attacks of abdominal pain or recurrent laryngeal edema [15]. Urticaria did not occur at any time in any of these patients. The skin swellings lasted 2 to 5 days; they affected mainly the extremities and the face, and the trunk less frequently. The abdominal attacks likewise lasted 2 to 5 days and were manifested as severe cramplike pains.

The clinical manifestation of hereditary angioedema type III is highly variable, and penetrance of the disease might be low; thus, we have observed obligate female carriers, even in their seventh decade, without any clinical symptoms [15,18]. Therefore, a considerable number of asymptomatic carriers may exist in the population.

Death by asphyxiation due to upper airway obstruction

In our patient series described in 2000 [15], one female had asphyxiated at the age of 16 during her first laryngeal edema attack. A second female asphyxiated at the age of 36 after 10 episodes of upper airway obstruction, and a third at the age of 38 during her eighth airway attack.

Onset of clinical symptoms

In our series of 36 patients [15], the onset of clinical symptoms ranged from the 1st to the 63rd year of life. In seven patients from four families, symptoms started before the age of 10 years. In 22 of the 36 females, the clinical symptoms began between the ages of 10 and 23, in 3 between the ages of 30 and 40, and in 4 between 47 and 63 years. In all patients the edema episodes occurred at irregular intervals, in most cases 3 to 12 times a year.

Potentially provoking factors

Exogenous estrogens

Oral contraceptives

In our first study [15], 10 of the 36 women with hereditary angioedema type III took estrogen-containing oral contraceptives and reported either the first appearance of clinical symptoms or a severe exacerbation of the disease in association with this treatment. In one female the skin swelling and abdominal symptoms appeared after starting the intake of oral contraceptives at the age of 18 and continued until the end of her second pregnancy at the age of 27. Since then, the patient has remained symptom-free for more than 15 years. Binkley and Davis reported two women who had swelling episodes after starting oral contraceptives [16]. Clinical symptoms were restricted to the time period of taking oral contraceptives. In the family reported by Martin and colleagues [17], four females had attacks of facial and acral edema, upper airway obstruction, and abdominal pain attacks (partly with ascites) after they took estrogens or during pregnancy. In 2003, data were presented concerning 39 women with HAE type III [18] who received oral contraceptives or estrogen replacement therapy. In 17 of the women, recurrent angioedema occurred for the first time after starting intake of oral contraceptives, and in 5 women a preexistent recurrent angioedema was exacerbated by oral contraceptives.

Estrogen replacement therapy

Binkley and Davis [16] gave an account of three females who had recurrent angioedema after starting estrogen replacement therapy. These females also had clinical symptoms during previous pregnancies but were symptom-free in the interval between pregnancies and onset of estrogen replacement therapy. In 2003, we described one woman from a family with HAE without C1-INH deficiency who experienced her first symptoms after onset of estrogen replacement therapy [18]. Furthermore, we cited three women whose symptoms were exacerbated by estrogen replacement therapy.

Pregnancies

One of our patients had relapsing skin swelling and abdominal pain attacks only during pregnancy. In another patient, skin swelling and abdominal attacks occurred after oral contraceptives were started and continued until the end of her second pregnancy [15]. Binkley and Davis [16] observed two patients who had clinical symptoms exclusively when pregnant. In three other women, symptoms were restricted to the periods of pregnancy and estrogen replacement therapy. Martin and colleagues noted four patients of one family who experienced edema episodes limited to times of oral contraceptive use or pregnancies [17].

Recurrent angioedema in women not taking oral contraceptives, receiving estrogen replacement therapy, or being pregnant

According to our study in 2000 [15], 24 patients in 10 families suffered from recurrent angioedema without receiving exogeneous estrogens (oral contraceptives or estrogen replacement therapy) or being pregnant. In the family described by Binkley and Davis [16], all seven affected women reported that their symptoms were restricted to the times of oral contraceptive use, estrogen replacement therapy, or pregnancy. Martin and colleagues reported on one woman who had clinical symptoms without taking oral contraceptives, receiving estrogen replacement therapy, or being pregnant [17]. In a later patient series, we reported that 15 (38%) of 39 patients with HAE type III angioedema received oral contraceptives or estrogen replacement therapy without experiencing angioedema symptoms. A similar percentage (37%) of women receiving hormone therapy without angioedema was demonstrated for patients with HAE type I [18].

Angiotensin-converting enzyme inhibitors

It is well known that ACE inhibitors are associated with the occurrence of angioedema in about 0.7% of individuals who receive this medication [21,22]. It has been reported that ACE inhibitors can induce an exacerbation of symptoms in patients with hereditary angioedema caused by C1 inhibitor deficiency [23]. We observed a 60-year-old man from a family with "hereditary angioedema with normal C1 inhibitor" who has had arterial hypertension since age 30 and was initially treated with hydrochlorothiazide and various β-receptor blockers [19]. The patient had four tongue swellings, one each in 1993, 1995, 1997, and 1999. Each swelling lasted for about 24 hours. Three of the swellings occurred 2 weeks after the patient had started taking a new antihypertensive drug (1993 and 1995, captopril; 1997, enalapril). The last episode, in 1999, occurred during the period from 1997 until now, when the patient received only hydrochlorothiazide and metoprolol. The patient has had no other symptoms of hereditary angioedema. Our observation demonstrates that ACE inhibitors might have a trigger function with regard to hereditary angioedema type III.

Angiotensin II type 1 receptor antagonists

Two unrelated patients with preexisting hereditary angioedema type III were described who experienced severe exacerbation of symptoms associated with using angiotensin II type 1 receptor antagonists [24]. A possible pathogenetic relationship between the underlying disease and the drug-associated angioedema was suggested.

The first patient was a 65-year-old woman, one of seven women in her family with recurrent angioedema and normal C1-inhibitor and C4. From ages 30 to 32 years, she had approximately 50 episodes of abdominal pain. An episode of facial swelling occurred at age 57 and again at age 61.

At age 63 she began treatment with losartan 50 mg/d for hypertension. Six months later she began to experience facial swelling—26 episodes in total within 17 months, with the final episodes occurring every 2 weeks. She received no other medication while taking losartan. After discontinuing losartan the patient has remained symptom-free for the past 18 months.

The second patient was a 70-year-old woman; she, as well as her daughter and granddaughter, had recurrent angioedema with normal C1 inhibitor and C4. Beginning at age 29, she had recurrent swelling of the tongue about five times a year. Approximately 10 episodes of facial swelling occurred from ages 29 to 40 years. At age 69, she began taking 80 mg of valsartan once daily for hypertension without any additional medication. Three weeks after starting treatment with valsartan, her angioedema attacks began to increase in frequency and severity; within the following 7 months, she had 10 episodes of facial swelling and 25 episodes of tongue swelling, 13 of which progressed to laryngeal edema. After discontinuing valsartan the patient has had no further swelling episodes for the past 9 months.

Of all the women reported to have hereditary angioedema type III that the author is aware of, the two patients described here are the only ones who received an angiotensin II receptor antagonist. Thus, these cases may indicate that patients with hereditary angioedema type III are at risk of severe exacerbation of their disease when exposed to this medication.

Laboratory results

In our study of 36 patients with HAE type III, laboratory results from the symptom-free intervals between edema attacks were available for 24 patients [15]. All patients had normal values for C1 inhibitor protein and activity and C4 concentration. In all patients with HAE type III, these tests were repeated two to five times at intervals of at least 2 months, and the results were confirmed consistently. In a subset of patients with HAE type III ($n = 9$), C1q was determined. All values were within normal range. In a further subset of the patients ($n = 14$), a variety of coagulation and fibrinolysis parameters in the symptom-free intervals were evaluated without evidence of activation. Specifically, thromboplastin time, activated partial thromboplastin time, fibrinogen, D-dimer, thrombin antithrombin complex, plasminogen, and antiplasmin plasmin complex were all within the normal range.

Laboratory results recorded from the acute edema episodes were obtained from 4 of the 26 patients originating from four different families. The four patients were tested during a total of eight acute attacks of skin swelling, one patient during an episode of abdominal swelling, and another during two laryngeal edema attacks. All patients had a normal plasma concentration of C1 inhibitor protein (mean 29 mg/dL; normal range (NR) = 15–35 mg/dL) and normal activity of plasma C1 INH (mean 94%; NR = 70%–130%) and C4 (mean 32 mg/dL; NR = 20–50 mg/dL).

Gender

The disease has been observed predominantly by far in women [15–18,20]. Fig. 2 shows a pedigree with affected women in four generations. In two families, however, the existence of clinically unaffected male carriers has been deduced [16,17]. Because all 76 patients from the initial studies cited above were women, it was assumed that the clinical phenotype might be limited to the female sex. However, in 2006 we described a family with dominantly inherited angioedema and normal C1 inhibitor in which not only five female but also three male family members were clinically affected [19]. Fig. 3 shows the family pedigree in which eight affected members are present in four successive generations. Laboratory results for five patients demonstrated normal values for C1 inhibitor activity and protein and C4 in plasma. Two of the three affected men have already died; however, reliable information about their clinical symptoms has been obtained through several other family members. The third affected man had three attacks when he was taking ACE inhibitors and one attack without such medication. Concerning the role of hormone medications, the initial manifestation of one woman's disease occurred 4 weeks after starting an oral contraceptive, whereas in another woman a remarkable improvement of symptoms was observed after she changed from an estrogen-containing contraceptive pill to a pill containing only a progestin.

In this family [19], women and men were clinically affected by recurrent angioedema. The familial angioedema observed by Gupta and colleagues

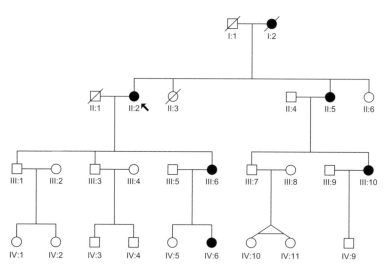

Fig. 2. Pedigree of a family with hereditary angioedema with normal C1 inhibitor. Six women from four generations are or were affected. The index patient is indicated by an arrow. ●, affected female; ○, unaffected female; □, unaffected male; ■, affected male; Slashed line, deceased family member.

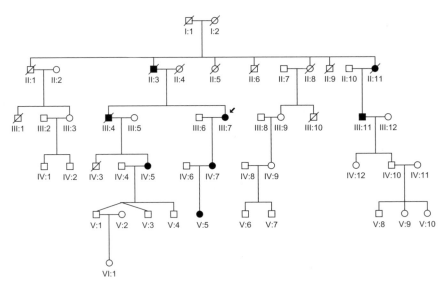

Fig. 3. Pedigree of a four-generation family with dominantly inherited angioedema with normal C1 inhibitor in which not only five females but also three male family members were clinically affected. The index patient is indicated by an arrow. ●, affected female; ○, unaffected female; □, unaffected male; ■, affected male; Slashed line, deceased family member.

[25] in three brothers appears to be HAE with normal C1 inhibitor in men; however, a possibly recessive inheritance pattern and a favorable response to treatment with antihistamines may indicate that the three brothers' condition is different from that of the family we observed [19]. In a study of 25 patients with idiopathic nonhistaminergic angioedema, Cicardi and colleagues [14] mentioned that four of these patients had affected relatives. In at least three of these families, all affected individuals were male. It is possible that these observations may be related to the type of HAE described in our family [19].

Inheritance

Within the families described in 2000 [15], between two and seven members per family were affected. In five families the disease had occurred in three successive generations and in the other five families in two successive generations. In two families we noted skipping, ie, one woman in each family transmitted the disease to offspring but showed no symptoms herself. When analyzing offspring of affected mothers including the last, often still disease-free generation, we counted in the pedigrees 27 males, 23 affected women and 17 unaffected women, resulting in a sex ratio (M:F) of 1:1.48. The presence of the disease in successive generations and the apparent male-to-male transmission [17] clearly favor the assumption of an autosomal dominant inheritance.

Genetic results

Normal C1 inhibitor activity and C4 in plasma were found in all patients; therefore, right from the beginning it seemed to be improbable that the cause of the disease would be a mutation in the C1 inhibitor gene. Binkley and Davis [16] found no abnormalities in either the 5' regulatory region or the coding sequences of the C1 inhibitor gene in affected individuals. In four of our affected patients we also looked for mutations in the C1 inhibitor gene and did not find any. Binkley and Davis also sequenced the 5' regulatory region of factor XII gene because it contains a known estrogen response element. However, they found no abnormalities in that region.

A recent genetic examination revealed new insight into HAE type III [20]. We hypothesized that an abnormal coagulation factor XII molecule may lead to inappropriate activation of the kinin-forming cascade of which factor XII is a major constituent [26]. Therefore, we performed a search for mutations in the factor XII (hageman factor) (*F12*) gene [20].

We studied 20 unrelated patients, all female and of German origin. All patients had experienced recurrent angioedema attacks, had one or more affected relatives (also exclusively women), and showed normal C1 inhibitor measurements. For several of these index patients, various numbers of family members could be included in the study.

The 14 exons and splice junctions of the *F12* gene [27] were screened in 20 unrelated patients by polymerase chain reaction (PCR) amplification and bidirectional sequencing. Aside from several known polymorphic variants, two different nonconservative missense mutations were identified in exon 9. Both mutations are located in exactly the same position, namely in the second position of the codon (ACG) encoding amino acid residue 309 of the mature protein, a threonine residue. "Mutation 1" (1032C→A), encountered in five unrelated patients, results in an AAG triplet encoding a lysine residue (Thr309Lys). "Mutation 2" (1032C→G), observed in one patient, predicts a threonine-to-arginine substitution (Thr309Arg). Thus, with respect to both mutations, the wild-type threonine residue is substituted by a basic amino acid residue. In accordance with the dominant inheritance pattern of the disease, patients are heterozygous for the respective mutations.

Neither of the two mutations was detected in 145 healthy control individuals in this control panel. Thus, missense mutations affecting Thr309 were seen in 6 of 20 patients, but in none of 145 controls ($P = .0000015$; Fisher's exact test).

In 6 of the 20 families, 23 individuals, all female, were clinically diagnosed with "hereditary angioedema with normal C1 inhibitor." Twenty-two of these women could be examined and were found to be heterozygous carriers of either the Thr309Lys or the Thr309Arg mutation. Two additional women carried the Thr309Lys mutation but have not experienced any angioedema symptoms up to now. Finally, there were eight male heterozygous carriers of a missense mutation of Thr309, all symptom-free [20].

Potential pathogenetic mechanisms

Hereditary angioedema type III is a rare disease that is characterized by recurrent angioedema and occurs mainly in women. It is not associated with a deficiency of C1 inhibitor activity.

Genetics

The results of our recent molecular genetic investigation revealed that HAE type III is not a homogeneous disease entity. Mutations in the *F12* gene were found in six families; however, the index patients of 14 other families did not show such mutations [20]. In the six families, the mutations of the *F12* gene were present in all affected women, in some of the men, and in some of the non-affected women (in whom clinical symptoms might occur in the future).

These results show that "hereditary angioedema with normal C1 inhibitor occurring mainly in women" (HAE type III) includes two or more conditions with different genetic causes. One of these conditions, "hereditary angioedema with coagulation factor XII gene mutations and normal C1 inhibitor," now has been identified [20].

Regarding both the patients and families in whom the present mutation screen remained negative, future studies will have to examine whether mutations eventually will be located within the noncoding regions of *F12* or whether other gene loci are involved.

Coagulation factor XII is a serine protease circulating in human plasma as a single-chain inactive zymogen at a concentration of approximately 30 μg/mL [27–29]. Upon contact with negatively charged surfaces, factor XII is activated by autoactivation and by plasma kallikrein, which itself is generated from prekallikrein by activated factor XII, high-molecular weight kininogen serving as a cofactor for reciprocal activation of factor XII and prekallikrein. Factor XII is a typical mosaic protein: following a leader peptide of 19 residues, the mature plasma protein consists of 596 amino acids and is organized in an N-terminal fibronectin type-II domain, followed by an epidermal growth factor–like domain, a fibronectin type-I domain, another epidermal growth factor–like domain, a kringle domain, a proline-rich region, and the C-terminal catalytic serine protease domain [28]. The amino acid substitutions described here are located in the poorly characterized proline-rich region of factor XII. This region appears to play some role in the binding of factor XII to negatively charged surfaces [29,30]. Thus, one may speculate that the mutations described by us [20] may influence mechanisms of contact activation and may eventually inappropriately facilitate factor XII activation.

The present findings are expected to have an immediate impact on the diagnostic evaluation and management of patients with recurrent angioedema but normal C1 inhibitor. Further studies will address, for example, the functional consequences of the described mutations, in particular with respect to kinin formation, the hormonal influence on trait expression, and the assumed genetic heterogeneity of hereditary angioedema with normal C1 inhibitor.

Reduced penetrance and sex-limited manifestation are well in agreement with previous clinical and pedigree observations [15,16]. It is known that the severity of clinical manifestation of hereditary angioedema with normal C1 inhibitor can vary widely, and that a large number of patients experience onset of symptoms only at an advanced age [15]. Thus, it seems possible that the two female mutation carriers mentioned above (their present ages being 16 years and 43 years, respectively) will still develop angioedema-related symptoms in the future.

Our data [20] demonstrate for the first time a highly significant relationship between a distinct human pathology—namely "hereditary angioedema with normal C1 inhibitor"—and mutations of the coagulation factor XII gene.

The predicted structural and functional impact of the mutations, their absence in healthy controls, and their cosegregation with the phenotype all provide strong support for the idea that these mutations cause disease. The remarkable observations that (1) two different mutations seen in patients but not controls both affect the identical DNA position, and (2) both lead to substitution of the wild-type threonine residue by a positively charged residue, lend further support to the assumption that these mutations play a disease-causing role.

Possible mediator responsible for angioedema formation

The mediator responsible for edema formation in hereditary angioedema type III is not known. However, consider the following facts: (1) there are many similarities concerning clinical symptoms of hereditary angioedema types I and III; (2) the percentages of women whose disease is negatively affected by estrogen-containing medications is similar in both conditions; (3) ACE inhibitors and angiotensin II type 1 receptor antagonists may lead to an increase in frequency and severity of attacks in HAE type III (according to the observations mentioned above) similar to HAE due to C1 inhibitor deficiency (HAE type I and II); and (4) the response to antihistamines and corticosteroids is lacking, at least in the patients reported up to now. These facts permit the speculation that edema formation in hereditary angioedema type III may also be related to the kinin pathway. It is possible that bradykinin is the most important mediator in HAE type III, similar to HAE types I and II.

Role of estrogens

In many women clinical symptoms either begin or are exacerbated following the intake of oral contraceptives or hormone replacement therapy, or during pregnancy. This observation has led to the assumption that the clinical manifestation of this new type of hereditary angioedema is estrogen-dependent. Binkley and Davis observed patients with typical symptoms of recurrent angioedema that were restricted to conditions of high estrogen levels; Binkley and Davis thereby created the (misleading) conception of an "estrogen-dependent" or "estrogen-associated" HAE [16,31,32]. In a recent analysis of 228 angioedema patients receiving oral contraceptives or hormone replacement therapy, it was demonstrated that in only 24 (62%) of 39 women with hereditary angioedema type III were the clinical symptoms induced or exacerbated after starting oral contraceptives or hormone replacement therapy; correspondingly, 15 (38%) of 39 women tolerated exogenous estrogens without any influence on their disease [18]. Almost identical numbers were observed with respect to women diagnosed with HAE due to C1 inhibitor deficiency. These results show that estrogens play a similar role in both conditions and that the negative influence of estrogens is not a specific sign for HAE type III [33]. Table 1 reveals, according to the information reported until now, that only in 16 of 81 women affected with HAE type III the attacks occurred exclusively during high estrogen level states ie, during pregnancy, during intake of oral contraceptives, or during estrogen replacement therapy. In the remaining 65 women the attacks occurred either independently of these states or they were present also before or after these states. In some of the patients the disease exacerbated during pregnancy, intake of oral contraceptives, or estrogen replacement therapy. Whether the influence of estrogen-containing oral contraceptives or hormonal

Table 1

Hereditary angioedema type III: Number of affected women reported until now, in whom the attacks occurred exclusively in high-estrogen states, ie, during pregnancy, intake of oral contraceptives, or estrogen replacement therapy

Authors	Reported families with HAE type III	Women affected with HAE type III	Women who had HAE attacks exclusively in high-estrogen states	Families in which all affected women had HAE attacks exclusively in high estrogen states
Bork et al, 2000 [15]	10	36	2	0
Binkley and Davis, 2000 [16]	1	7	7	1
Martin et al, 2001 [17]	1	4	3	0
Bork et al, 2003 [18]	10	29	4	0
Bork et al, 2006 [19]	1	5	0	0
Total	23	81	16	1

replacement therapy on the kinin pathway actually plays a role in favoring angioedema formation in patients with hereditary angioedema is far from being clear today. The observations available until now suggest that even among patients with underlying hereditary angioedema, administration of estrogen does not always result in the appearance or worsening of symptoms. Other factors that might predispose women with angioedema to new or exacerbated symptoms when treated with estrogens could include, for example, a functionally or quantitatively relevant genetic polymorphism in the kinin system. Information about such polymorphisms might be important in identifying women whose angioedema would be aggravated by administration of estrogen-containing medications.

Role of ACE inhibitors and angiotensin II type 1 receptor antagonists

ACE inhibitors and angiotensin II type 1 receptor antagonists may lead to an increase in the frequency and severity of attacks in HAE III, according to the observations mentioned above. Concerning ACE inhibitors, HAE type III shares this feature with HAE due to C1 inhibitor deficiency. This state of affairs points to an important role of bradykinin in the pathogenesis of HAE type III.

Affected males

Our observation of a family with affected women and men [19] can be interpreted in two ways: men, although having the same genetic defect, might have a highly reduced chance for clinical manifestation of angioedema, because of either the lack of female-specific risk factors (for example, estrogen-containing medications or pregnancy) or the presence of male-specific protective factors; eventually, manifestation may need a further triggering factor. Such a factor could be either endogenous—for example, a certain genetic cofactor—or exogenous, such as treatment of hypertension with ACE inhibitors, as in one of the patients [19].

Alternatively, one may speculate that this family represents another disease entity with a different underlying defect, namely hereditary angioedema with normal C1 inhibitor, but not restricted to the female sex. The identification of further underlying molecular defects in this and other families with hereditary angioedema type III will allow researchers to define various potentially existing forms of hereditary angioedema with normal C1 inhibitor.

Diagnosis

Up to now the clinical diagnosis of "hereditary angioedema with normal C1 inhibitor" has required that patients have the above-mentioned clinical symptoms, one or more family members also affected with these symptoms, the exclusion of familial and hereditary chronic urticaria with urticaria-associated angioedema, and normal C1 inhibitor activity and protein in plasma. The diagnosis "hereditary angioedema with coagulation factor XII gene mutation" requires the corresponding demonstration of the mutation.

Management

Danazol

One of our patients had frequent skin swellings and abdominal pain attacks and received a daily, oral dose of 100 mg danazol. Under this treatment the patient became symptom-free for 9 years. Then the treatment with danazol was discontinued to see whether the patient could do without it. Two weeks later an exacerbation with skin swellings and bowel angioedema occurred. Therefore, 4 weeks later treatment with danazol was resumed; the symptoms have not recurred since then (7 years as of now). Another patient received 100 mg danazol per day for 2 weeks and later on 200 mg daily for an additional 4 months without any therapeutic effect [15]. Martin and colleagues [17] reported one patient whose symptoms improved when she was treated with danazol 200 mg every other day. The dosage was progressively tapered to 200 mg/week without relapse after 2.5 years. Herrmann and colleagues [34] described a 31-year-old woman who suffered from HAE with normal C1 inhibitor. They initially treated the patient with 600 mg danazol daily. No further attacks occurred subsequently; the dosage of danazol was reduced at 2-week intervals to 100 mg daily and then over subsequent weeks to 50 mg twice weekly. At the latter dose the patient has been free of symptoms for more than 2 years. Side effects included an initial weight gain of around 8 kg, a mild papulopustulous acne, and amenorrhea.

Tranexamic acid

Two patients were treated with the antifibrinolytic agent tranexamic acid, 1 g three times a day for 4 months, without any success [15].

C1 inhibitor concentrate

Four women having 11 episodes of acute laryngeal edema had received 1000-U doses of C1 inhibitor concentrate (Berinert P, ZLB Behring, Germany) [15]. This treatment had proven ineffective.

Corticosteroids and antihistamines

In 23 of our patients, previous edema attacks had been treated by antihistamines and corticosteroids (at a dosage of 100 to 250 mg one or more times daily). This treatment had been ineffective in all 23 cases [15]. Likewise, the patient cited by Herrmann and colleagues did not respond to corticosteroids and antihistamines [34].

References

[1] Greaves M, Lawlor F. Angioedema: manifestations and management. J Am Acad Dermatol 1991;25:155–65.

[2] Champion RH, Roberts OB, Carpenter RG, et al. Urticaria and angioedema: a review of 554 patients. Br J Dermatol 1969;81:588–97.

[3] Agostoni A, Cicardi M. Hereditary and acquired C1-inhibitor deficiency: biological and clinical characteristics in 235 patients. Medicine (Baltimore) 1992;71:206–15.

[4] Bork K, Siedlecki K, Bosch S, et al. Asphyxiation by laryngeal edema in patients with hereditary angioedema. Mayo Clin Proc 2000;75:349–54.

[5] Giannoccaro PJ, Wallace GJ, Higginson LAJ, et al. Fatal angioedema associated with enalapril. Can J Cardiol 1989;5:335–6.

[6] Ulmer JL, Garvey MJ. Fatal angioedema associated with lisinopril. Ann Pharmacother 1992;26:1245–6.

[7] Jason DR. Fatal angioedema associated with captopril. J Forensic Sci 1992;37:1418–21.

[8] Oike Y, Ogata Y, Higashi D, et al. Fatal angioedema associated with enalapril. Intern Med 1993;32:308–10.

[9] Dean DE, Schultz DL, Powers RH. Asphyxia due to angiotensin converting enzyme (ACE) inhibitor mediated angioedema of the tongue during the treatment of hypertensive heart disease. J Forensic Sci 2001;46:1239–43.

[10] Landerman NS, Webster ME, Becker EL, et al. Hereditary angioneurotic edema: II. Deficiency of inhibitor for serum-globulin permeability factor and/or plasma kallikrein. J Allergy 1962;33:330–41.

[11] Donaldson VH, Evans RR. A biochemical abnormality in hereditary angioneurotic edema: absence of serum inhibitor of C1-esterase. Am J Med 1963;35:37–44.

[12] Alsenz J, Bork K, Loos M. Autoantibody-mediated acquired deficiency of C1 inhibitor. N Engl J Med 1987;316:1360–6.

[13] Jackson J, Sim RB, Whelan A, et al. An IgG autoantibody which inactivates C1-inhibitor. Nature 1986;323:722–4.

[14] Cicardi M, Bergamaschini L, Zingale LC, et al. Idiopathic nonhistaminergic angioedema. Am J Med 1999;106:650–4.

[15] Bork K, Barnstedt S, Koch P, et al. Hereditary angioedema with normal C1- inhibitor activity in women. Lancet 2000;356:213–7.

[16] Binkley KE, Davis A III. Clinical, biochemical, and genetic characterization of a novel estrogen-dependent inherited form of angioedema. J Allergy Clin Immunol 2000;106: 546–50.

[17] Martin L, Degenne D, Toutain A, et al. Hereditary angioedema type III: an additional French pedigree with autosomal dominant transmission. J Allergy Clin Immunol 2001; 107:747–8.

[18] Bork K, Fischer B, Dewald G. Recurrent episodes of skin angioedema and severe attacks of abdominal pain induced by oral contraceptives or hormone replacement therapy. Am J Med 2003;114:294–8.

[19] Bork K, Gül D, Dewald G. Hereditary angio-oedema with normal C1 inhibitor in a family with affected women and men. Br J Dermatol 2006;154:542–5.

[20] Dewald G, Bork K. Missense mutations in the coagulation factor XII (Hageman factor) gene in hereditary angioedema with normal C1 inhibitor. Biochem Biophys Res Commun 2006; 343:1286–9.

[21] Sabroe RA, Black AK. Angiotensin-converting enzyme (ACE) inhibitors and angio-oedema. Br J Dermatol 1997;136:153–8.

[22] Vleeming W, van Amsterdam JGC, Stricker BHC, et al. ACE inhibitor-induced angioedema. Drug Saf 1998;18:171–88.

[23] Agostoni A, Cicardi M. Contraindications to the use of ACE inhibitors in patients with C1 esterase inhibitor deficiency. Am J Med 1991;90:278.

[24] Bork K, Dewald G. Hereditary angioedema type III, angioedema associated with angiotensin II receptor antagonists, and female sex. Am J Med 2004;116:644–5.

[25] Gupta S, Yu F, Klaustermeyer WB. New-variant hereditary angioedema in three brothers with normal C1 esterase inhibitor level and function. Allergy 2004;59:557–8.

[26] Kaplan AP, Joseph K, Shibayama Y, et al. The intrinsic coagulation/kinin-forming cascade: Assembly in plasma and cell surfaces in inflammation. Adv Immunol 1997;66:225–72.

[27] Cool DE, MacGillivray RTA. Characterization of the human blood coagulation factor XII gene. Intron/exon gene organization and analysis of the 5′-flanking region. J Biol Chem 1987;262:13662–73.

[28] Cool DE, Edgell CJ, Louie GV, et al. Characterization of human blood coagulation factor XII cDNA. Prediction of the primary structure of factor XII and the tertiary structure of beta-factor XIIa. J Biol Chem 1985;260:13666–76.

[29] Citarella F, Aiuti A, La Porta C, et al. Control of human coagulation by recombinant serine proteases. Blood clotting is activated by recombinant factor XII deleted of five regulatory domains. Eur J Biochem 1992;208:23–30.

[30] Citarella F, Ravon DM, Pascucci B, et al. Structure/function analysis of human factor XII using recombinant deletion mutants. Evidence for an additional region involved in the binding to negatively charged surfaces. Eur J Biochem 1996;238:240–9.

[31] Binkley KE, Davis AE III. Estrogen-dependent inherited angioedema. Transfus Apheresis Sci 2003;29:215–9.

[32] Binkley KE, Davis AE III. Estrogen-dependent and estrogen-associated inherited angioedema (previously HAE III). J Allergy Clin Immunol 2004;114(3 Suppl):S62–4.

[33] Bork K, Fischer B. Influence of oral contraceptives or hormonal replacement therapy on hereditary forms of recurrent angioedema. J Allergy Clin Immunol 2004;114(3 Suppl):S85–8.

[34] Herrmann G, Schneider L, Krieg T, et al. Efficacy of danazol treatment in a patient with the new variant of hereditary angio-oedema (HAE III). Br J Dermatol 2004;150:157–8.

ELSEVIER
SAUNDERS

Immunol Allergy Clin N Am
26 (2006) 725–737

IMMUNOLOGY
AND ALLERGY
CLINICS
OF NORTH AMERICA

Angiotensin-Converting Enzyme Inhibitor-Associated Angioedema

James Brian Byrd, MD[a], Albert Adam, PhD[b],
Nancy J. Brown, MD[a],*

[a]Division of Clinical Pharmacology, Vanderbilt University School of Medicine,
560 Robinson Research Building, Nashville, TN 37232-6602, USA
[b]Faculty of Pharmacy, University of Montreal, 2900 boulevard Édouard-Montpetit,
C.P. 6128 Succursale Centre-Ville, Montréal, Québec H3C 3J7, Canada

Angiotensin-converting enzyme (ACE, kininase II) inhibitors reduce mortality in patients who have hypertension, congestive heart failure, and diabetic nephropathy and in patients who are at high risk for cardiovascular events [1–4]. ACE inhibitor–associated angioedema is a rare, potentially life-threatening side effect of treatment with ACE inhibitors. Reactions range from mild swelling of the tongue, lips, other areas of the face, hands, feet, or bowel to life-threatening airway compromise. Given that 35 to 40 million people worldwide are currently taking ACE inhibitors, the number of people at risk for this side effect is substantial.

Clinical features of angiotensin-converting enzyme inhibitor–associated angioedema

Angioedema is characterized by self-limited, nonpitting edema of vascular origin. The most common sites of involvement in ACE inhibitor–associated angioedema are the lips, tongue, and face (Fig. 1) [5–7]. Pruritis and urticaria, seen in hypersensitivity reactions, typically do not accompany ACE inhibitor–associated angioedema. Rarely, ACE inhibitor–associated angioedema may involve the bowel wall [8]. In such cases, patients present with nausea and vomiting, abdominal pain, diarrhea, or ascites associated with ACE inhibitor use. The diagnosis may be confirmed by the

This work was supported by NIH Grants HL079184 and HL076133 and National Center for Research Resources Grant RR-00095.

* Corresponding author.
E-mail address: nancy.j.brown@vanderbilt.edu (N.J. Brown).

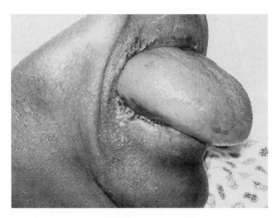

Fig. 1. Photograph illustrating a case of ACE inhibitor–associated angioedema. (*From* Agah R, Bandi V, Guntupalli KK. Angioedema: the role of ACE inhibitors and factors associated with poor clinical outcome. Intensive Care Med 1997;23(7):795; with permission.)

identification of bowel edema on CT scan and resolution of symptoms with discontinuation of ACE inhibitor use; however, failure to suspect ACE inhibitor–associated angioedema can lead to surgical procedures. A unique form of hemioral angioedema has been associated with tissue-type plasminogen activator administration in stroke patients who are taking an ACE inhibitor [9].

The incidence of ACE inhibitor–associated angioedema is highest during the first month of treatment. Slater and colleagues [10] reported a 14-fold higher incidence of angioedema during the first week of treatment compared with subsequent exposure, and Kostis and colleagues [7] observed that the incidence of angioedema was ninefold higher in the first month of ACE inhibitor use. Although the risk for angioedema per exposure is greatest in the first month of treatment with an ACE inhibitor, the majority of cases occur after 1 month of treatment, and as many as 27% of cases present more than 6 months after initiation of ACE inhibitor therapy [11,12]. The range of treatment duration before angioedema onset was 1 day to 10 years in one series [13].

Early recognition and discontinuation of the ACE inhibitor remain the primary therapy for ACE inhibitor–associated angioedema. To date, no other specific treatment for ACE inhibitor–associated angioedema has been tested in clinical trials. Nielsen and Gramstad [14] reported that administration of complement 1 inhibitor (C1-INH) concentrate decreased symptoms in a patient who had ACE inhibitor–associated angioedema. Administration of fresh frozen plasma has also been effective in the treatment of resistant cases [15]. Although bradykinin receptor antagonism has proved effective in shortening the duration of hereditary angioedema [16], clinical trials of bradykinin receptor antagonism in ACE inhibitor–associated angioedema are lacking. Primary supportive therapy includes management of the airway, with a minority of cases requiring intubation or cricothyroidotomy. Although many physicians treat patients with antihistamines, steroids, and, in more severe cases, epinephrine, no clinical trial has addressed the efficacy of these treatments in ACE inhibitor–associated angioedema. Patients presenting with angioedema should be tested for C1 inhibitor function as well as C4, C3, and C1q antigens to exclude the possibility of hereditary angioedema or acquired C1-INH deficiency.

The adverse event of angioedema is a class effect of ACE inhibitors, so patients who have experienced angioedema while taking one ACE inhibitor may not be treated with another. Because it may be desirable to substitute another drug that interrupts the renin-angiotensin system for an ACE inhibitor in patients who have experienced angioedema, Cicardi and colleagues [6] addressed the safety of administering an angiotensin receptor blocker (ARB) to patients who have previously experienced ACE inhibitor–associated angioedema. This study suggests that it is generally safe to treat individuals who have a history of ACE inhibitor–associated angioedema with an ARB. Unlike ACE inhibitors, ARBs do not potentiate the vasodilator response to the vasoactive peptide bradykinin [17]. However, studies in animals suggest that ARBs may increase bradykinin by means of the actions of angiotensin II at the unblocked angiotensin II type 2 receptor [18]. In addition, circulating bradykinin concentrations may be increased in individuals who are taking an ARB [19]. Although case reports suggest that patients taking ARBs occasionally experience angioedema, the rate of angioedema in patients taking ARBs is not increased over that observed in the general public, and it is significantly lower than the rate of angioedema observed during ACE inhibition [20].

Epidemiology of angiotensin-converting enzyme inhibitor–associated angioedema

The reported incidence of ACE inhibitor–associated angioedema varies from 0.1% to 0.7%, calculated from postmarketing surveillance or epidemiologic studies, to as great as 2.8% to 6% when ascertained prospectively in clinical trials [10,21,22]. Black Americans have an incidence of ACE inhibitor–associated angioedema that is four to five times that of white Americans [7,12,23]. Smoking, increasing age, and female gender are also associated with increased risk for ACE inhibitor–associated angioedema, whereas diabetics appear to be protected from ACE inhibitor–associated angioedema (Table 1) [7,22,24]. A history of ACE inhibitor–associated cough increases the risk for ACE inhibitor–associated angioedema [24]. However, patterns of racial differences in the incidence of ACE inhibitor–associated cough and ACE inhibitor–associated angioedema do not suggest a tight link between cough and angioedema. For example, Asians frequently develop cough but are not at increased risk for angioedema [24,25]. At least one group has reported an increased rate of ACE inhibitor–associated angioedema among immunocompromised cardiac and renal transplant patients [26].

Table 1
Risk factors associated with angioedema in the Omapatrilat Cardiovascular Treatment versus Enalapril (OCTAVE) study

Risk factor	Odds ratio (95% CI)	P value
African American race	2.97 (2.24, 3.92)	<.0001
Current smoker	2.49 (1.86, 3.34)	<.0001
Female gender	1.49 (1.16, 1.91)	.002
Seasonal allergies	1.52 (1.12, 2.06)	.008
Former smoker	1.47 (1.09, 1.99)	.013
History of diabetes	0.58 (0.38, 0.90)	.014

Data from Bristol Myers Squibb Co., New York, NY.

Mechanisms of angiotensin-converting enzyme inhibitor–associated angioedema

The mechanism or mechanisms of ACE inhibitor–associated angioedema remain to be elucidated, but the clinical presentation of ACE inhibitor–associated angioedema may provide clues to its causation. As noted earlier, ACE inhibitor–associated angioedema frequently occurs after prolonged exposure; furthermore, it may remit spontaneously and recur after prolonged time intervals [27]. This pattern excludes a typical allergic or immediate hypersensitivity mechanism and suggests that some concurrent event or exposure must precipitate angioedema in an individual who is taking an ACE inhibitor. In this regard, ACE inhibitor–associated angioedema resembles hereditary angioedema, or C1 esterase inhibitor deficiency, in which patients also report recurrent episodes.

ACE inactivates bradykinin, and studies using bradykinin receptor antagonists demonstrate that endogenous bradykinin contributes to the hypotensive effects of ACE inhibitors [28]. Activation of the kallikrein-kinin system, with consumption of kininogen, has been demonstrated in patients who have hereditary angioedema [29]. In addition, genetic bradykinin receptor deficiency attenuates edema in C1 esterase–deficient mice [30]. Bradykinin B_1 and B_2 receptors are expressed in the tongue, laryngeal areas, and parotid gland [31]. Administration of the bradykinin receptor antagonist Icatabant (HOE 140, JE 049) decreases the severity of hereditary angioedema in Phase II trials [16].

Although the role of the kallikrein-kinin system in the pathogenesis of hereditary angioedema is established, definitive data implicating bradykinin in ACE inhibitor–associated angioedema are sparse. Nussberger and coworkers [32] reported that circulating bradykinin concentrations were increased in both patients who had hereditary angioedema and in one patient who had ACE inhibitor–associated angioedema; however, bradykinin concentrations in control subjects taking ACE inhibitors without angioedema [33] were not reported in this study. In addition, although high molecular weight kininogen is consumed in hereditary forms of angioedema, there is no increased cleavage of kininogen in ACE inhibitor–associated angioedema [33]. This observation is compatible with the hypothesis that, to the extent that bradykinin plays a role in ACE inhibitor–associated angioedema, impaired metabolism, rather than increased generation, contributes to this adverse event.

Animal models of angioedema

In addition to bradykinin, substance P is another peptide substrate of ACE that causes vasodilation and increased vascular permeability. Both bradykinin and substance P produce tracheal edema in animals [34,35]. For example, Emanueli and coworkers [34] demonstrated that acute administration of captopril or enalapril caused extravasation of Evans blue dye in the trachea, stomach, duodenum, and pancreas of mice. Pretreatment with either the bradykinin B_2 receptor antagonist HOE 140 or the substance P (tachykinin) neurokinin I (NK1) receptor antagonist SR 140,333 significantly decreased ACE inhibitor–induced plasma extravasation. Genetic disruption of the B_2 receptor also prevented ACE inhibitor–induced edema. Taken together, these data suggest that ACE inhibition causes edema by increasing tissue bradykinin, which in turn can stimulate substance P release from nerve fibers, leading to enhanced vascular permeability and leakage of plasma protein into the interstitial space [36,37]. It follows that enzymes involved in the degradation of either bradykinin or substance P may be involved in the pathogenesis of ACE inhibitor–associated angioedema in specific populations.

Angiotensin-converting enzyme inhibitors and the degradation of vasoactive peptides

Fig. 2 shows the enzymatic pathways involved in the degradation of the ACE substrates bradykinin and substance P. Bradykinin is degraded primarily by ACE (Enzyme Classification [EC] 3.4.15.1); however, during ACE inhibition, other enzymes, including neutral endopeptidase (NEP-24.11, EC 3.4.24.11), aminopeptidase P (APP, EC 3.4.11.9), and kininase I (carboxypeptidase N, EC 3.4.17.3), assume greater importance in the metabolism of bradykinin [38]. Cleavage of bradykinin by kininase I yields the active metabolite des-Arg^9-bradykinin, which is inactivated primarily by APP.

To determine whether impaired metabolism of kinins contributes to the pathogenesis of angioedema in the presence of ACE inhibition, Blais and colleagues [39] characterized the ex vivo metabolism of bradykinin in the sera of patients who had a history of ACE inhibitor–associated angioedema. In the absence of ACE inhibition, kininase I played a minor role in degradation of bradykinin. During ACE inhibition, the relative contribution of kininase I to the degradation of bradykinin increased to a greater extent in individuals who had a history of angioedema compared with normal controls. This finding of enhanced degradation of bradykinin by means of kininase I during ACE inhibition in the sera of individuals who have ACE

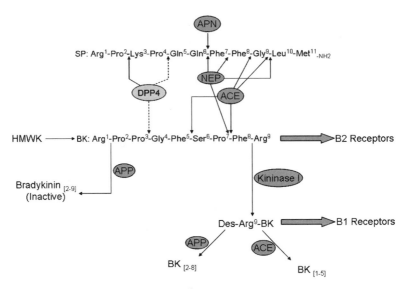

Fig. 2. Degradation of bradykinin, des-Arg^9-bradykinin, and substance P. APN, aminopeptidase N or M; APP, aminopeptidase P; BK, bradykinin; DPP4, dipeptidyl peptidase IV; HMWK, high molecular weight kininogen; NEP, neutral endopeptidase; SP, substance P.

inhibitor–associated angioedema suggests that such individuals may have a defect in a non-ACE, non–kininase I pathway of kinin degradation.

Aminopeptidase P deficiency and adverse events associated with angiotensin-converting enzyme inhibition

During ACE inhibition, the contribution of APP to the degradation of bradykinin also increases [40,41]. Thus, during ACE inhibition, deficient APP activity could lead to enhanced degradation of bradykinin by means of kininase I, as well as to accumulation of bradykinin and des-Arg^9-bradykinin. Adam and coworkers [42] have reported decreased APP activity in sera from 39 patients (20 male, 19 female; 16 ± 10 nmol/min/mL) who had a history of ACE inhibitor–associated angioedema compared with 39 age- and gender-matched hypertensive controls (23 ± 10 nmol/min/mL; $P = .003$). No difference was found between groups in kininase I activity in the absence of ACE inhibition.

The investigators further characterized the metabolism of bradykinin and des-Arg^9-bradykinin following stimulation of the formation of bradykinin ex vivo by incubation of plasma with glass beads. In the presence of ACE inhibition (enalaprilat 130 nM), there was a slight but significant ($P = .022$) decrease in the catabolism of bradykinin in patients who had a history of angioedema (Fig. 3), compared with controls. However, there was no difference between angioedema patients and controls in maximal bradykinin concentration or area under the curve (AUC). In contrast, both maximal

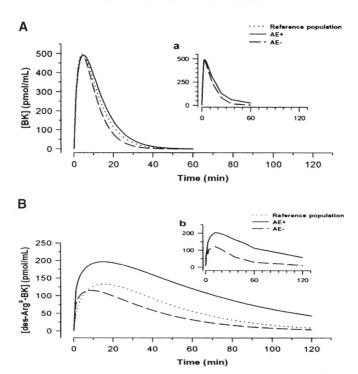

Fig. 3. Model-fitted profiles of the formation of bradykinin (BK) (*A*) and des-Arg^9-bradykinin (des-Arg^9-BK) (*B*) in individuals who have a history of angioedema (AE+, *solid lines*) and controls (AE−, *dashed lines*) after activation of the contact system in the presence of enalaprilat with glass beads. Dotted lines are for a reference population. Superscript graphs show measured values. (*From* Molinaro G, Cugno M, Perez M, et al. Angiotensin-converting enzyme inhibitor–associated angioedema is characterized by a slower degradation of des-arginine(9)-bradykinin. J Pharmacol Exp Ther 2002;303(1):234; with permission.)

des-Arg^9-bradykinin concentration and the AUC for des-Arg^9-bradykinin were significantly increased in patients who had angioedema, as was the half-life of degradation. These data confirm that des-Arg^9-bradykinin formation by kininase I is increased in the sera of patients who have angioedema (again, suggesting a defect in other degradative pathways of bradykinin) and raise the possibility that des-Arg^9-bradykinin degradation is decreased.

Despite these intriguing data, decreased APP activity does not account entirely for the pathophysiology of ACE inhibitor–associated angioedema. One third of the individuals with a history of ACE inhibitor–associated angioedema who were studied by Adam and co-workers [42] had normal APP activity. In addition, the frequency of decreased APP activity in the population (18%) exceeds the incidence of angioedema in ACE inhibitor–exposed patients [43]. Moreover, the investigators have not found a decrease in APP activity or des-Arg^9-bradykinin metabolism in black individuals who have a history of ACE inhibitor–associated angioedema [39,44]. Taken together, these data suggest that other pathways may play a role in ACE inhibitor–associated angioedema.

Dipeptidyl peptidase IV and angiotensin-converting enzyme inhibitor–associated angioedema

In addition to increasing vascular permeability directly by means of its B_2 receptor, bradykinin stimulates the release of substance P, which causes increased vascular permeability by acting at the NK_1 receptor [37]. ACE also degrades substance P; however, in the setting of ACE inhibition, dipeptidyl peptidase IV (DPPIV/CD26; EC 3.4.14.5) sequentially degrades substance P to substance P 5-11, which lacks vasoactive function and is susceptible to further degradation by aminopeptidase N (APN/CD13, 3.4.11.2) [45]. LeFebvre and colleagues reported decreased DPPIV activity in a small number of patients who had a history of ACE inhibitor–associated angioedema [46]. The group has recently confirmed this finding in a larger group of patients (abstract). Interestingly, clinical risk factors for angioedema, including increasing age and smoking [24], were associated with decreased DPPIV antigen concentrations in this study.

Pharmacogenetics of angiotensin-converting enzyme inhibitor–associated angioedema

In contrast to hereditary angioedema, in which mutations in the C1 esterase gene have been identified, ACE inhibitor–associated angioedema results, by definition, after an environmental exposure and must involve gene–environment interactions. The heritability of ACE inhibitor–associated angioedema has not been formally established. However, ethnic differences in the frequency of angioedema provide presumptive evidence that genetic factors play a role.

Efforts to identify genetic factors predisposing to ACE inhibitor–associated angioedema have focused on enzymes involved in the degradation of bradykinin and substance P. For example, based on data indicating that APP activity is decreased in patients who have angioedema, Duan and colleagues [44] performed quantitative trait locus analysis to determine the genetic factors regulating APP activity in eight pedigrees in which at least one family member had developed an anaphylactoid reaction during hemodialysis (six families), angioedema (one family), or both (one family) (Fig. 4). Human APP exists in two forms, a glycosylphosphatidylinositol (GPI) anchored membrane form (hmAPP) and a cytosolic form (hcAPP). The gene encoding hmAPP (*XPNPEP2*, MIM 300,145) localizes to chromosome Xq26.1 [47], whereas the gene encoding hcAPP (*XPNPEPL*, MIM 602,443) localizes to 10q25.1 [48]. Duan and colleagues [44] found that variation in the *XPNPEP2* gene accounted for 34% of the heritability of plasma APP activity. There was no linkage with the hcAPP gene, suggesting

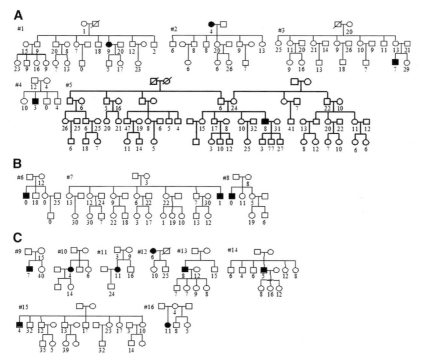

Fig. 4. Pedigrees including a proband (*shaded*) with hemodialysis-induced anaphylactoid reaction during ACE inhibitor use. The proband in family 8 had angioedema; the proband in family 3 had both an anaphylactoid reaction during hemodialysis and angioedema. Numbers indicate individual APP activities. □ male with no history of angioedema or anaphylactoid reaction; ■ male affected by angioedema and/or anaphylactoid reaction; ○ female with no history of angioedema or anaphylactoid reaction; ● female affected by angioedema and/or anaphylactoid reaction. (*From* Duan QL, Nikpoor B, Dube MP, et al. A variant in XPNPEP2 is associated with angioedema induced by angiotensin I–converting enzyme inhibitors. Am J Hum Genet 2005;77(4):619; with permission.)

that hmAPP is the primary contributor to plasma APP activity. The investigators identified a single nucleotide polymorphism (C-2399A) that associated with plasma APP activity, such that the A allele was associated with lower APP activity. An association between the C-2399A genotype and APP activity as well as angioedema was confirmed in unrelated white ACE inhibitor–associated angioedema cases and controls. In addition, the investigators identified a 175bp genomic deletion (g.2953-3127) that resulted in a truncated mAPP protein in one family with a proband who had both angioedema and an anaphylactoid reaction to hemodialysis. The mutant protein lacked both predicted active sites and the GPI anchor.

Despite this interesting finding that variation in the gene encoding mAPP predicted APP activity in families who had a history of anaphylactoid reactions, the applicability of these findings to prediction of those who are at greatest risk for ACE inhibitor–associated angioedema is not certain. Although individuals who have anaphylactoid reactions may experience angioedema, these reactions are typically characterized by hypotension, which is not a feature of ACE inhibitor–associated angioedema. In addition, mutations in an X-linked gene are not likely to account for the majority of cases of angioedema, given that angioedema affects women more often than men.

Brown and coworkers have recently studied the relationship between polymorphisms in the gene encoding DPPIV and ACE inhibitor–associated angioedema. Human DPPIV is located on chromosome 2 locus 2q24.3 and contains 26 exons [49]. Using single-strand conformational polymorphism, the authors identified 17 polymorphisms in the gene. One of these, a synonymous single nucleotide polymorphism T24C, correlated with DPPIV antigen and activity concentrations in white individuals, suggesting that it is in linkage disequilibrium with an as yet unidentified functional polymorphism. Whether the frequency of the allele associated with lower DPPIV antigen concentrations is increased in individuals who have a history of ACE inhibitor–associated angioedema is under investigation.

Future directions

Ultimately, verification of a role for bradykinin, substance P, or any other vasoactive peptide substrate of ACE in the pathogenesis of ACE inhibitor–associated angioedema will require clinical studies assessing the effect of specific peptide receptor antagonists on the resolution of angioedema. Such studies are difficult to conduct because of the remitting and relapsing pattern of ACE inhibitor–associated angioedema. Drugs that inhibit DPPIV are currently under development for the treatment of diabetes, and clinical studies using these drugs may serve to clarify the role of DPPIV in the pathogenesis of ACE inhibitor–associated angioedema. Finally, the development of animal models of ACE inhibitor–associated angioedema would greatly enhance our ability to study the causation of this adverse drug effect.

References

[1] The SOLVD investigators. Effect of enalapril on survival in patients with reduced left ventricular ejection fractions and congestive heart failure. N Engl J Med 1991;325:293–302.

[2] Lewis EJ, Hunsicker LG, Bain RP, et al. The effect of angiotensin-converting-enzyme inhibition on diabetic nephropathy. The Collaborative Study Group. N Engl J Med 1993;329:1456–62.

[3] Yusuf S, Sleight P, Pogue J, et al. Effects of an angiotensin-converting-enzyme inhibitor, ramipril, on cardiovascular events in high-risk patients. The Heart Outcomes Prevention Evaluation Study Investigators. N Engl J Med 2000;342(3):145–53.

[4] Dahlof B, Sever PS, Poulter NR, et al. Prevention of cardiovascular events with an antihypertensive regimen of amlodipine adding perindopril as required versus atenolol adding

bendroflumethiazide as required, in the Anglo-Scandinavian Cardiac Outcomes Trial—Blood Pressure Lowering Arm (ASCOT-BPLA): a multicentre randomised controlled trial. Lancet 2005;366(9489):895–906.

[5] Agah R, Bandi V, Guntupalli KK. Angioedema: the role of ACE inhibitors and factors associated with poor clinical outcome. Intensive Care Med 1997;23(7):793–6.

[6] Cicardi M, Zingale LC, Bergamaschini L, et al. Angioedema associated with angiotensin-converting enzyme inhibitor use: outcome after switching to a different treatment. Arch Intern Med 2004;164(8):910–3.

[7] Kostis JB, Kim HJ, Rusnak J, et al. Incidence and characteristics of angioedema associated with enalapril. Arch Intern Med 2005;165(14):1637–42.

[8] Schmidt TD, McGrath KM. Angiotensin-converting enzyme inhibitor angioedema of the intestine: a case report and review of the literature. Am J Med Sci 2002;324(2):106–8.

[9] Hill MD, Buchan AM. Thrombolysis for acute ischemic stroke: results of the Canadian Alteplase for Stroke Effectiveness Study. CMAJ 2005;172(10):1307–12.

[10] Slater EE, Merrill DD, Guess HA, et al. Clinical profile of angioedema associated with angiotensin converting-enzyme inhibition. JAMA 1988;260(7):967–70.

[11] Gabb GM, Ryan P, Wing LM, et al. Epidemiological study of angioedema and ACE inhibitors. Aust N Z J Med 1996;26(6):777–82.

[12] Brown NJ, Ray WA, Snowden M, et al. Black Americans have an increased rate of angiotensin converting enzyme inhibitor–associated angioedema. Clin Pharmacol Ther 1996;60(1):8–13.

[13] Agostoni A, Cicardi M, Cugno M, et al. Angioedema due to angiotensin-converting enzyme inhibitors. Immunopharmacology 1999;44(1–2):21–5.

[14] Nielsen EW, Gramstad S. Angioedema from angiotensin-converting enzyme (ACE) inhibitor treated with complement 1 (C1) inhibitor concentrate. Acta Anaesthesiol Scand 2006;50(1):120–2.

[15] Warrier MR, Copilevitz CA, Dykewicz MS, et al. Fresh frozen plasma in the treatment of resistant angiotensin-converting enzyme inhibitor angioedema. Ann Allergy Asthma Immunol 2004;92(5):573–5.

[16] Icatibant. HOE 140, JE 049, JE049. Drugs R D 2004;5(6):343–8.

[17] Cockcroft JR, Sciberras DG, Goldberg MR, et al. Comparison of angiotensin-converting enzyme inhibition with angiotensin II receptor antagonism in the human forearm. J Cardiovasc Pharmacol 1993;22(4):579–84.

[18] Carey RM, Wang ZQ, Siragy HM. Role of the angiotensin type 2 receptor in the regulation of blood pressure and renal function. Hypertension 2000;35(1 Pt 2):155–63 [Review. 92 refs.].

[19] Campbell DJ, Krum H, Esler MD. Losartan increases bradykinin levels in hypertensive humans. Circulation 2005;111(3):315–20.

[20] Johnsen SP, Jacobsen J, Monster TB, et al. Risk of first-time hospitalization for angioedema among users of ACE inhibitors and angiotensin receptor antagonists. Am J Med 2005;118(12):1428–9.

[21] Sica DA. The African American Study of Kidney Disease and Hypertension (AASK) trial: what more have we learned? J Clin Hypertens (Greenwich) 2003;5(2):159–67.

[22] Kostis JB, Packer M, Black HR, et al. Omapatrilat and enalapril in patients with hypertension: the Omapatrilat Cardiovascular Treatment vs. Enalapril (OCTAVE) trial. Am J Hypertens 2004;17(2):103–11.

[23] Gibbs CR, Lip GY, Beevers DG. Angioedema due to ACE inhibitors: increased risk in patients of African origin. Br J Clin Pharmacol 1999;48(6):861–5 [see comments].

[24] Morimoto T, Gandhi TK, Fiskio JM, et al. An evaluation of risk factors for adverse drug events associated with angiotensin-converting enzyme inhibitors. J Eval Clin Pract 2004;10(4):499–509.

[25] Woo KS, Norris RM, Nicholls G. Racial difference in incidence of cough with angiotensin-converting enzyme inhibitors (a tale of two cities). Am J Cardiol 1995;75(14):967–8.

[26] Abbosh J, Anderson JA, Levine AB, et al. Angiotensin converting enzyme inhibitor–induced angioedema more prevalent in transplant patients. Ann Allergy Asthma Immunol 1999; 82(5):473–6.

[27] Brown NJ, Snowden M, Griffin MR. Recurrent angiotensin-converting enzyme inhibitor–associated angioedema. JAMA 1997;278(3):232–3.

[28] Gainer JV, Morrow JD, Loveland A, et al. Effect of bradykinin-receptor blockade on the response to angiotensin-converting-enzyme inhibitor in normotensive and hypertensive subjects. N Engl J Med 1998;339(18):1285–92.

[29] Schapira M, Silver LD, Scott CF, et al. Prekallikrein activation and high-molecular-weight kininogen consumption in hereditary angioedema. N Engl J Med 1983;308:1050–4.

[30] Han ED, MacFarlane RC, Mulligan AN, et al. Increased vascular permeability in C1 inhibitor–deficient mice mediated by the bradykinin type 2 receptor. J Clin Invest 2002;109(8): 1057–63.

[31] Moreau ME, Dubreuil P, Molinaro G, et al. Expression of metallopeptidases and kinin receptors in swine oropharyngeal tissues: effects of angiotensin I–converting enzyme inhibition and inflammation. J Pharmacol Exp Ther 2005;315(3):1065–74.

[32] Nussberger J, Cugno M, Amstutz C, et al. Plasma bradykinin in angio-oedema. Lancet 1998; 351(9117):1693–7.

[33] Molinaro G, Cugno M, Perez M, et al. Angiotensin-converting enzyme inhibitor-associated angioedema is characterized by a slower degradation of des-arginine(9)-bradykinin. J Pharmacol Exp Ther 2002;303(1):232–7.

[34] Emanueli C, Grady EF, Madeddu P, et al. Acute ACE inhibition causes plasma extravasation in mice that is mediated by bradykinin and substance P. Hypertension 1998;31(6): 1299–304.

[35] Sulpizio AC, Pullen MA, Edwards RM, et al. The effect of acute angiotensin-converting enzyme and neutral endopeptidase 24.11 inhibition on plasma extravasation in the rat. J Pharmacol Exp Ther 2004;309(3):1141–7.

[36] Kopp UC, Farley DM, Smith LA. Bradykinin-mediated activation of renal sensory neurons due to prostaglandin-dependent release of substance P. Am J Physiol 1997;272(6 Pt 2): R2009–16.

[37] Campos MM, Calixto JB. Neurokinin mediation of edema and inflammation. Neuropeptides 2000;34(5):314–22.

[38] Moreau ME, Garbacki N, Molinaro G, et al. The kallikrein-kinin system: current and future pharmacological targets. J Pharmacol Sci 2005;99(1):6–38.

[39] Blais CJ, Rouleau JL, Brown NJ, et al. Serum metabolism of bradykinin and des-Arg9-bradykinin in patients with angiotensin-converting enzyme inhibitor–associated angioedema. Immunopharmacology 1999;43(2–3):293–302.

[40] Ersahin C, Simmons WH. Inhibition of both aminopeptidase P and angiotensin-converting enzyme prevents bradykinin degradation in the rat coronary circulation. J Cardiovasc Pharmacol 1997;30(1):96–101.

[41] Kim KS, Kumar S, Simmons WH, et al. Inhibition of aminopeptidase P potentiates wheal response to bradykinin in angiotensin-converting enzyme inhibitor–treated humans. J Pharmacol Exp Ther 2000;292(1):295–8.

[42] Adam A, Cugno M, Molinaro G, et al. Aminopeptidase P in individuals with a history of angio-oedema on ACE inhibitors. Lancet 2002;359(9323):2088–9.

[43] Cyr M, Lepage Y, Blais C Jr, et al. Bradykinin and des-Arg(9)-bradykinin metabolic pathways and kinetics of activation of human plasma. Am J Physiol Heart Circ Physiol 2001; 281(1):H275–83.

[44] Duan QL, Nikpoor B, Dube MP, et al. A variant in XPNPEP2 is associated with angioedema induced by angiotensin I–converting enzyme inhibitors. Am J Hum Genet 2005;77(4): 617–26.

[45] Russell JS, Chi H, Lantry LE, et al. Substance P and neurokinin A metabolism by cultured human skeletal muscle myocytes and fibroblasts. Peptides 1996;17(8):1397–403.

[46] Lefebvre J, Murphey LJ, Hartert TV, et al. Dipeptidyly peptidase IV activity in patients with ACE-inhibitor—associated angioedema. Hypertension 2002;39:460–4.

[47] Sprinkle TJ, Stone AA, Venema RC, et al. Assignment of the membrane-bound human aminopeptidase P gene (XPNPEP2) to chromosome Xq25. Genomics 1998;50(1):114–6.

[48] Sprinkle TJ, Caldwell C, Ryan JW. Cloning, chromosomal sublocalization of the human soluble aminopeptidase P gene (XPNPEP1) to 10q25.3 and conservation of the putative proton shuttle and metal ligand binding sites with XPNPEP2. Arch Biochem Biophys 2000;378(1): 51–6.

[49] Abbott CA, Baker E, Sutherland GR, et al. Genomic organization, exact localization, and tissue expression of the human CD26 (dipeptidyl peptidase IV) gene. Immunogenetics 1994;40(5):331–8.

ELSEVIER
SAUNDERS

Immunol Allergy Clin N Am
26 (2006) 739–751

IMMUNOLOGY
AND ALLERGY
CLINICS
OF NORTH AMERICA

Idiopathic Recurrent Angioedema

Evangelo Frigas, MD*, Miguel Park, MD

*Division of Allergic Disease and Internal Medicine, Mayo Clinic College of Medicine,
200 First Street SW, Rochester, MN 55905, USA*

Angioedema is a constellation of syndromes characterized by swelling of the deeper layers of the skin or submucosa (or both). Although any part of the body may be affected by angioedema, the face and extremities are most commonly involved. The swellings develop from extravasation of plasma in the affected areas. The extravasation is due to transient increase in endothelial permeability caused by vasoactive substances produced locally. Episodic abdominal pain arising from swelling of the submucosa of any portion of the gastrointestinal tract may occur without swelling of the skin; therefore, angioedema should be included in the differential diagnosis of intermittent, unexplained abdominal pain.

In some cases of angioedema, it has been shown that the extravasation of plasma is caused by vasoactive substances secreted from activated mast cells and eosinophils or by inappropriate activation of the complement and kinin systems, which may be either hereditary or acquired. However, in most clinical presentations of angioedema, the pathogenetic mechanism is unknown. About 50% of the cases of angioedema are accompanied by urticaria and pruritus.

The diagnosis of idiopathic recurrent angioedema is made after a comprehensive evaluation has ruled out the known causes of angioedema. Currently, the prevalence, natural history, and prognostic variables of idiopathic recurrent angioedema are unknown.

Taking a comprehensive personal and family history, performing a physical examination, and compulsively monitoring the response to therapy are the most beneficial and cost-effective diagnostic and treatment tools. All patients with idiopathic recurrent angioedema should be reevaluated once a year or more often if deemed necessary by their primary care physicians,

This work was supported by an educational and research fund from Mayo Clinic College of Medicine, Grant No. ZZ0551.

* Corresponding author.
E-mail address: frigas.evangelo@mayo.edu (E. Frigas).

with the intent of identifying the pathogenesis and optimizing treatment. Diligent and knowledgeable follow-up spares patients costly or unnecessary tests and ineffective or harmful treatment. This is best achieved by close collaboration between the patient's primary care physician and an allergist or dermatologist in an academic medical center that has a clinical, research, and education program in angioedema where innovative treatments and research protocols may be used effectively and safely for the patient. Currently, the treatment of idiopathic recurrent angioedema with or without urticaria is difficult and frustrating for patients and their physicians because it is often only partially effective and is labor-intensive, lengthy, and expensive.

The term angioedema is used to define a localized, sudden, transient, and often recurrent swelling of the skin or submucosa (or both). It is caused by vasoactive substances that produce a transient increase in endothelial permeability [1,2]. In the skin, the nonpitting swellings are accompanied by the cardinal signs of inflammation, namely, rubor and calor, whereas dolor and functio laesa appear when angioedema involves the throat or gastrointestinal tract [3]. These swellings usually last from a couple of hours to a few days and resolve spontaneously. About 50% of cases are accompanied by urticaria and pruritus [3].

The term idiopathic recurrent angioedema is used when three or more episodes of angioedema have occurred within a period of 6 months to 1 year without any cause being identified after an initial comprehensive medical evaluation and periodic reevaluations and treatment trials. This category of angioedema is not only the most common of the cases of recurrent angioedema referred to a tertiary medical center, but it is also among the most distressing for the patient and the most challenging for the medical profession. In our experience, the amplified morbidity from severity and chronicity of symptoms, secondary chronic anxiety, depression, and side effects of the medications used for treatment requires a systematic and comprehensive approach. An essential component of this approach is close collaboration between the patient's primary care physician and a specialist in allergy or dermatology who practices in a tertiary referral medical center that has a program in patient care, education, and research in angioedema. This approach best addresses the needs of these patients for periodic reevaluation in search of the pathogenesis, the effectiveness of the therapy used, careful and safe testing of innovative treatments, and research protocols.

The purpose of this manuscript is to share our experience in the Urticaria/Angioedema Clinic at Mayo Clinic in the care of patients with idiopathic recurrent angioedema and to review the literature on the subject.

Epidemiology

The epidemiology of idiopathic recurrent angioedema is not well known. For the past 50 years, it generally has been reported that urticaria, angioedema, or both, will affect 10% to 20% of people worldwide at least once in their lifetime [4]. Women are affected slightly more often than men, and at presentation 50% of patients are found to have both urticaria and angioedema [4]. In a recent study of 107 patients with chronic urticaria, angioedema occurred much more often, affecting 83% of the patients studied [5]. With regard to the etiology, it has been reported and reiterated in a recent symposium on urticaria and angioedema that most of the cases are idiopathic [6,7].

Clinical presentations and endoscopic and radiographic findings

Angioedema of the skin is typically nonpitting, with ill-defined margins. The skin is swollen, tender, and warm. Frequently, a burning sensation is described by patients, and pruritus is present when there is urticaria. Attacks of recurrent angioedema may last from hours to a few days and usually resolve spontaneously [3]. Occasionally, physical trauma or stress may be the precipitating factor. Angioedema may affect any part of the gastrointestinal tract. Angioedema of the wall of the bowel may cause obstruction as well as nausea, vomiting, and abdominal pain.

The radiographic findings in angioedema of the gastrointestinal tract may consist of dilated loops of bowel, obliteration of the normal contour of the mucosa, "thumbprinting sign," narrowing of the lumen, and ascites [3]. Unless there is a high degree of awareness of patients who present repeatedly to an emergency department with recurrent abdominal pain without angioedema of the skin, the diagnosis of gastrointestinal angioedema is easily missed [3]. The abdominal symptoms from recurrent angioedema may be attributed to anxiety and somatization, which may lead to a psychiatric evaluation. Fever and leukocytosis are unusual in recurrent angioedema. Cases of cerebral angioedema leading to migraine and transient ischemic attacks have been described [8].

There are no distinguishing radiologic or endoscopic findings that may differentiate idiopathic, recurrent angioedema from any of the other categories of chronic recurrent angioedema. Angioedema due to hereditary deficiency of the C1 esterase inhibitor is not accompanied by urticaria and pruritus.

Pathogenesis

Excessive production or decreased catabolization of molecules that increase vascular permeability cause extravasation of plasma under the skin or the submucosa, and this produces the swellings of angioedema. The best known and most frequently cited vasoactive molecules are histamine, tryptase, prostaglandin $F_{2\alpha}$ from mast cells, and bradykinin from inappropriate and excessive activation of the complement and kallikrein systems [1–3,9,10].

Food allergens (especially shellfish, nuts, and peanuts), latex, and insect venoms as well as several medications can release histamine from sensitized mast cells and may produce angioedema on an IgE-mediated basis. Some medications (narcotics, polymyxin, d-tubocurarine) may cause angioedema owing to their ability to cause direct mast cell degranulation in the absence of IgE antibodies against the drug. Nonsteroidal anti-inflammatory drugs, oral contraceptives, and estrogen replacement medications have all been associated with angioedema, although the mechanisms of their effects have not been clearly established [2,3,9]. Angiotension II inhibitors, such as losartan and angiotensin-converting enzyme (ACE) inhibitors, such as captopril, can cause angioedema in a subset of patients taking these drugs [2,3,9]. Angioedema develops in 1% to 5% of patients who take ACE inhibitors, and it is indistinguishable from any other form of angioedema [2,3]. Although most cases of angioedema caused by ACE inhibitors occur during the first week of therapy, symptoms of angioedema have occurred after a patient has taken the medication for several years [2,3]. It has been proposed that ACE-induced angioedema may be caused by either an increase in the production of bradykinin [9,10] or a decrease in its catabolization [1].

In susceptible persons, physical agents such as cold, pressure, vibration, and ultraviolet radiation can produce angioedema, which usually is associated with urticaria [11]. The ice-cube test is used to rule out a cold-induced pathogenesis. Cold-induced angioedema and urticaria have been reported in association with cryoglobulins, cold agglutinin disease, cryofibrinogenemia, and paroxysmal cold hemoglobinuria [12].

The pathogenetic mechanisms of recurrent angioedema from inherited and acquired deficiencies of the C1 esterase inhibitor of the complement and kallikrein systems have been well studied. In these categories of angioedema, the swellings are suspected to be due to increased local production of various kinins, especially bradykinin and kallidin [2,3,13] (see article by Davis elsewhere in this issue).

About 20 years ago, it was first reported that occasionally autoimmune thyroid disease, recurrent angioedema, and urticaria are associated [14]. Consequently, antithyroid autoantibodies, such as the antimicrosomal and antithyroglobulin autoantibodies associated with Hashimoto thyroiditis, were singled out as a possible autoimmune cause in a subset of patients with angioedema and urticaria [15]. Gruber and colleagues [16] proposed that possibly anti-IgE autoantibodies have a role in autoimmune urticaria and angioedema, and Grattan and colleagues [17] researched the identification of these autoantibodies by performing an autologous skin test. They reported a 30% incidence of positive skin test reactions in patients with chronic urticaria [17]. Hide and colleagues [18] published evidence of a histamine-releasing IgG anti–high-affinity IgE receptor (anti-FcεR1) autoantibody and proposed it as a cause for autoimmune urticaria and angioedema. The presence of IgG autoantibodies in the sera of certain patients with chronic urticaria against the alpha chain of FcεR1 has been confirmed by others as well [19–23]. According to this autoimmune model, the patho-genetic mechanism is mediated by specific IgG autoantibodies that bind and cross-link adjacent FcεR1 receptors or the Fc portion of adjacent IgE mol-ecules, leading to mast cell activation and the release of vasoactive sub-stances that cause angioedema or urticaria (or both). In this pathogenetic model, a synchronous activation of the complement system with the produc-tion of C5a may augment the reaction in some patients [24,25].

Most recently, it has been reported that normal serum has a natural auto-antibody (anti-FcεRia) against the α subunit of the IgE receptor [26,27]. It has been hypothesized that through an abnormal control mechanism these anti-receptor autoantibodies may lead to mast cell activation and development of angioedema [26,27]. Yet another autoimmune model has been suggested that does not involve immunoglobulins, in which the release of vasoactive me-diators in patients with idiopathic chronic urticaria and angioedema may be mediated by aberrant regulation of the intracellular signal transduction of the p21ras pathway [28]. An autoimmune model for the pathogenesis of angioe-dema appears to be supported by reports on the benefits of plasmapheresis in patients with severe chronic urticaria [29], on intravenous immunoglobulin for chronic autoimmune urticaria [30], on cyclosporine for chronic idiopathic urticaria [31], and on methotrexate for chronic idiopathic urticaria [32].

In summary, the pathogenesis of idiopathic recurrent angioedema with or without urticaria is not known. The great variety of clinical presentations and the large number of patients with angioedema recalcitrant to therapy suggest that the pathophysiologic mechanisms are more complex than has been reported. Multicenter, large, double-blind, placebo-controlled clinical studies with well-selected patients may provide reliable and useful informa-tion on the treatment of idiopathic recurrent angioedema.

Initial evaluation, diagnosis, and differential diagnosis at an allergy specialty clinic

All patients who have chronic recurrent angioedema (ie, three or more episodes within 3 to 6 months) with or without chronic urticaria or who have recurrent abdominal pain that is unexplained after adequate evaluation and treatment by their primary care physician or gastroenterologist should have a work-up for angioedema by a specialist, usually an allergist or der-matologist. On the basis of our experience, we propose the algorithm in Fig. 1 for the systematic evaluation of patients with recurrent angioedema with or without urticaria. In the Urticaria/Angioedema Clinic, which was established in the Division of Allergic Diseases and Internal Medicine at Mayo Clinic Rochester in 1995, we evaluate approximately 300 to 400 patients annually, most of them referred by their primary care physicians.

Our work-up often consists of a comprehensive physical examination, a detailed personal and family history, and skin biopsy for standard light microscopic direct and indirect immunofluorescence when needed, especially

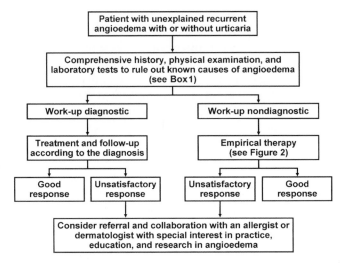

Fig. 1. Proposed algorithm for the evaluation and follow-up of patients with recurrent angioedema.

if there is coexisting urticaria or if vasculitis is suspected. The importance of a comprehensive general medical evaluation for these patients cannot be overemphasized. As appreciated by others, the benefits from the history and physical examination outweigh the contribution of laboratory tests [33]. Special attention must be directed to confirming the patient's description of symptoms and time course. Is what the patient describes as swelling angioedema? Carefully look for any relationship between the patient's symptoms and activities, eating, and medication use. Is the patient's angioedema caused by medications taken? The inquiry about medications used by the patient should include asking about over-the-counter preparations, herbs, vitamins, and supplements, which patients often do not consider as medications and therefore do not mention them unless asked. Often, this relationship between medication and angioedema is not self-evident. Discontinuation of the medication(s) may be necessary to clear this possibility. In addition to the medications, any skin products and cosmetics used by the patient must be identified. The initial work-up includes the following laboratory tests: complement C4, C1q, CH50, C1 esterase inhibitor by functional and quantitative assays, and a panel for mast cell-mediator screening, which includes measurements of tryptase and calcitonin in the serum and histamine, N-methylhistamine, and prostaglandin $F_{2\alpha}$ in a 24-hour urine collection. The following are also part of the work-up if they have not been performed recently: a complete blood count, chemistry group, serum protein electrophoresis, total serum IgE, erythrocyte sedimentation rate, and a thyroid cascade, which includes testing for antithyroid antibodies. When warranted by the patient's history, allergy skin tests or specific IgE blood tests are performed to rule out latex and food allergy.

In our experience, the most common initial diagnosis is idiopathic recurrent angioedema with or without urticaria, for which antihistamine therapy prescribed by the referring physicians usually has been partially beneficial. Almost all the patients report a beneficial effect from treatment with systemic glucocorticoids, but the beneficial effect vanishes as soon as the glucocorticoid therapy is stopped. Some patients are not able to discontinue the glucocorticoid therapy because of intolerable angioedema, urticaria, and pruritus. We have not identified the large number of patients with recurrent angioedema due to C1 esterase inhibitor deficiency that authors from other tertiary medical centers have reported [34]. Also, we have not encountered the high incidence of angioedema reported to be caused by oral contraceptives, estrogen replacement therapy, ACE inhibitors, and associated autoimmune thyroid disease [5,35–37]. Annually, about 1% of the patients we evaluate have swelling that masquerades as angioedema, such as allergic or contact dermatitis, folliculitis, cellulitis, acne rosacea associated with lymphedema, angioedema associated with eosinophilic panniculitis [38], idiopathic cyclic edema, angioedema associated with hypereosinophilia [39], granulomatous cheilitis, and superior vena cava syndrome.

Since we started testing with the panel for mast cell mediators in the late 1990s, we have found several patients with chronic idiopathic recurrent angioedema with or without urticaria who have an isolated elevation of prostaglandin $F_{2\alpha}$ in the urine but normal levels of the other mediators. These patients are not atopic and have no clinical evidence of localized or systemic mastocytosis. The biopsy of the bone marrow is normal and there is no increase in the number of mast cells. In our experience, these patients may benefit from treatment with aspirin. We have also noted that the increase in prostaglandin $F_{2\alpha}$ in the urine returns to normal after aspirin has been added to their treatment.

After the initial clinical evaluation and laboratory work-up, the patient's case is assigned to one of the diagnostic categories listed in Box 1. The diagnosis of idiopathic recurrent angioedema is the most common. Whenever possible, these patients are scheduled for reevaluation in 3 to 4 months, or more often if necessary, with 30-minute visits to determine whether any new symptoms warrant further investigation and to reappraise the benefits and side effects of therapy. Furthermore, once a year, a general medical examination is repeated with the same components as described above to search for the pathogenesis and to reassess the effectiveness of therapy. We have found that frequent communication and supportive collaboration among the specialist, patient, and patient's primary care physician are essential for the success of the treatment.

Treatment

Treatment and follow-up depend on the diagnosis. Angioedema caused by medications, allergens, or physical agents is treated by eliminating the

---

Box 1. Diagnostic categories of recurrent angioedemas

Idiopathic angioedemas with or without urticaria (the most
    common category)
Medication induced
Allergen induced
Physically induced
Associated with autoimmune disease of the thyroid
Combination of 2 or more of the above
From deficiency of C1 esterase inhibitor of the complement and
    kallikrein systems (C1 INH)
Hereditary C1 INH deficiency
Variant 1: 80%–85% of cases of hereditary angioedema
Variant 2: 10%–15% of cases of hereditary angioedema
Variant 3: percentage of cases of hereditary angioedema
    unknown
Acquired with C1 INH deficiency
Variant 1: associated with malignancies, mainly
    lymphoproliferative
Variant 2: caused by anti–C1 INH autoantibodies
Pseudoangioedemas

---

causative agent. Hereditary angioedema, which often requires lifelong treatment and careful monitoring, is best treated by referral to a specialist in the management of this disease. Idiopathic, chronic, recurrent angioedema may require treatment and follow-up for several years. Depending on where the patient lives and the resources available in the area, the best care is provided by effective collaboration between the patient's primary care physician and a specialist in a clinic with a program for treatment, education, and research in angioedema and urticaria. In our Urticaria/Angioedema Clinic, we offer patient education, treatment, and research studies.

    For general patient education, patients with idiopathic angioedema are given the same instructions as for other categories of angioedema and urticaria. Specifically, patients are given instructions for skin care, primarily the avoidance of dryness. Patients are advised to avoid cosmetic creams, perfumes, and deodorants when these items are suspected to cause flares of symptoms. They also are advised to avoid any medication that has caused or is suspected to cause an exacerbation of their symptoms. Often this information is not self-evident to patients. For example, patients sensitive to aspirin may use a product that contains aspirin; thus, these patients should be given a list of commonly used products and medications containing aspirin. Other factors reviewed with patients are diet, exercise, and stress. Patients with a history of angioedema of the throat are provided with an action plan to use in case of recurrence. This includes instructions on how to use epinephrine, systemic glucocorticoids, and antihistamines; wearing an identification bracelet; and telephone numbers for immediate access to care.

For medications, we often follow a stepwise ladder approach as shown in Fig. 2. The benefit of antihistamine therapy for patients with idiopathic angioedema varies, but these medications are almost always helpful. In step 1, we usually start with a nonsedating or less-sedating antihistamine, such as fexofenadine, cetirizine, loratadine, or desloratadine, taken during the daytime. Often, as has been reported, we have found off-label dosage beneficial, especially when there is coexisting urticaria [2]. For example, we have prescribed fexofenadine 180 mg, cetirizine 10 mg, or loratadine 10 mg twice daily instead of once daily with good results, provided the agent is needed, well tolerated, and does not interfere with the other medications the patient is taking. If this treatment is not satisfactory, we proceed with step 2 by adding a sedating antihistamine such as doxepin, hydroxyzine, or diphenhydramine, usually taken at bedtime. The dose of the sedating antihistamine should be titrated according to its effectiveness in controlling the patient's symptoms, provided of course it is well tolerated and does not interfere with the rest of the medications the patient is taking. For example, we have often noted the need for increasing the nightly dose of doxepin from 10 mg up to 150 mg to adequately control the patient's symptoms. We have also noted that increasing the dose of doxepin above 150 mg adds no further improvement in symptom control. Other authors have reported very good results with higher doses of sedating antihistamine (specifically diphenhydramine) taken during the daytime [2]. They have noted that the patient's sedation and somnolence from diphenhydramine wears off after 1 week of treatment [2]. They also noted benefit from combining H_1 with H_2 antihistamines and a leukotriene antagonist [2].

When the antihistamine therapy in step 2 is only partially effective (often the case for our patients with idiopathic angioedema), we proceed with step 3, in which, in addition to the antihistamines, we prescribe treatment trials with other medications we or others have found helpful in this setting. Review of the literature shows that patients with severe angioedema with or without urticaria that is not responding to antihistamine therapy have

		Additional medications (see text)
	Sedating antihistamine	Sedating antihistamine
Nonsedating antihistamine	Nonsedating antihistamine	Nonsedating antihistamine
Step 1	**Step 2**	**Step 3**

Fig. 2. Algorithm for a stepwise ladder approach in the treatment of angioedema with or without urticaria. For detailed description of the medications used in steps 1, 2, and 3, see the text in the "Treatment" section.

been treated with a wide variety of medications. In a double-blind random-ized study, cyclosporine was found to be effective in patients with chronic idiopathic urticaria and angioedema [31]. Our experience with cyclosporine has been limited because of concerns about the potential for severe side effects and the benefit often encountered with drugs with fewer side effects. In another double-blind randomized study, nifedipine was found to be ben-eficial for patients with chronic idiopathic urticaria and angioedema [40]. In the few cases in which we have tried this medication, we have not noticed benefit. Other reported beneficial therapies include methotrexate [32,41], androgens with impeded androgenic action [42,43], and warfarin [44].

In our experience, treatment trials for 2 to 4 months with either colchicine 0.6 mg once or twice daily [45] or dapsone 25 mg twice daily and titrated up to 100 mg twice daily [46], or sulfasalazine 500 mg once or twice daily are often helpful [47,48]. We rule out glucose-6-phosphate dehydrogenase defi-ciency before initiation of therapy with dapsone. We also have noted benefit occasionally with recombinant interferon α. We usually start at a dose of 3 million units subcutaneously 3 times weekly. At times, the addition of indo-methacin (sustained release) 75 mg once or twice daily to the treatment with dapsone or interferon has been beneficial in improving the control of symp-toms. We evaluate the benefit from any of the medication trials mentioned above after 2 to 4 months. During these trials, we closely monitor the patients with office visits and laboratory testing every 2 to 3 weeks to ensure there are no side effects from the treatment. In a subset of patients with id-iopathic recurrent angioedema and increased urinary levels of prostaglandin $F_{2\alpha}$, we have noted benefit from adding aspirin to the treatment at any of the steps described above, provided the patients are not sensitive to aspirin. We usually start with 81 mg of aspirin, and if needed and tolerated by the pa-tient, we gradually increase the dosage up to 1.5 to 2 g per day in divided doses.

Systemic glucocorticoids, although very effective for the majority of patients with recurrent angioedema, in our experience should not be used long-term because of their cumulative and severe side effects and the fre-quent development of dependence. Therefore, we use them sparingly and only in short courses (ie, prednisone 20 mg for 5 to 7 days usually without tapering), for treatment of protracted attacks of angioedema or after epi-nephrine has been used to treat a severe attack of angioedema or urticaria.

Summary

The treatment of idiopathic, chronic, recurrent angioedema with or with-out urticaria is difficult, both for patients and their physicians, because treat-ment often is only partially effective and is labor-intensive, expensive, and lengthy. New medications for urticaria and angioedema that currently are being tested clinically may prove effective.

Acknowledgments

The authors thank LaDonna G. Mourning for secretarial assistance with rough drafts and the typing of the manuscript. Editing, proofreading, and reference verification were provided by the Section of Scientific Publications, Mayo Clinic.

References

[1] Cugno M, Nussberger J, Cicardi M, et al. Bradykinin and the pathophysiology of angioedema. Int Immunopharmacol 2003;3(3):311–7.

[2] Kaplan AP, Greaves MW. Angioedema. J Am Acad Dermatol 2005;53(3):373–88.

[3] Frigas E, Nzeako UC. Angioedema. Pathogenesis, differential diagnosis, and treatment. Clin Rev Allergy Immunol 2002;23(2):217–31.

[4] Mathews KP. Urticaria and angioedema. J Allergy Clin Immunol 1983;72(1):1–14.

[5] Beltrani VS. Angioedema: some "new" thoughts regarding idiopathic angioedema. In: Greaves MW, Kaplan AP, editors. Urticaria and angioedema. New York: Marcel Dekker; 2004. p. 421–39.

[6] Champion RH, Greaves MW, Black AK, et al. The urticarias. Edinburgh: Churchill Livingstone; 1985.

[7] Champion RH. Urticaria: then and now. Br J Dermatol 1988;119(4):427–36.

[8] Krause KH, Rentrop U, Mehregan U. Cerebral manifestations in angioneurotic edema. J Neurol Sci 1979;42(3):429–35 [in German].

[9] Pellacani A, Brunner HR, Nussberger J. Plasma kinins increase after angiotensin-converting enzyme inhibition in human subjects. Clin Sci (Lond) 1994;87(5):567–74.

[10] Nussberger J, Cugno M, Cicardi M. Bradykinin-mediated angioedema. N Engl J Med 2002; 347(8):621–2.

[11] Casale TB, Sampson HA, Hanifin J, et al. Guide to physical urticarias. J Allergy Clin Immunol 1988;82(5 Pt 1):758–63.

[12] Gorevic PD. Cryopathies: cryoglobulins and cryofibrinogenemia. In: Frank MM, Austen KF, Claman HN, et al, editors. Samter's immunologic diseases. 5th edition vol 2. Boston: Little, Brown and Company; 1995. p. 951–74.

[13] Nzeako UC, Frigas E, Tremaine WJ. Hereditary angioedema: a broad review for clinicians. Arch Intern Med 2001;161(20):2417–29.

[14] Leznoff A, Josse RG, Denburg J, et al. Association of chronic urticaria and angioedema with thyroid autoimmunity. Arch Dermatol 1983;119(8):636–40.

[15] Leznoff A, Sussman GL. Syndrome of idiopathic chronic urticaria and angioedema with thyroid autoimmunity: a study of 90 patients. J Allergy Clin Immunol 1989;84(1):66–71.

[16] Gruber BL, Baeza ML, Marchese MJ, et al. Prevalence and functional role of anti-IgE autoantibodies in urticarial syndromes. J Invest Dermatol 1988;90(2):213–7.

[17] Grattan CE, Hamon CG, Cowan MA, et al. Preliminary identification of a low molecular weight serological mediator in chronic idiopathic urticaria. Br J Dermatol 1988;119(2): 179–83.

[18] Hide M, Francis DM, Grattan CE, et al. Autoantibodies against the high-affinity IgE receptor as a cause of histamine release in chronic urticaria. N Engl J Med 1993;328(22):1599–604.

[19] Fiebiger E, Maurer D, Holub H, et al. Serum IgG autoantibodies directed against the α chain of FcεRI: a selective marker and pathogenetic factor for a distinct subset of chronic urticaria patients? J Clin Invest 1995;96(6):2606–12.

[20] Fiebiger E, Hammerschmid F, Stingl G, et al. Anti-FcεRIα autoantibodies in autoimmune-mediated disorders: identification of a structure-function relationship. J Clin Invest 1998; 101(1):243–51.

[21] Niimi N, Francis DM, Kermani F, et al. Dermal mast cell activation by autoantibodies against the high affinity IgE receptor in chronic urticaria. J Invest Dermatol 1996;106(5): 1001–6.

[22] Ferrer M, Kinet JP, Kaplan AP. Comparative studies of functional and binding assays for IgG anti-FcεRIα (α-subunit) in chronic urticaria. J Allergy Clin Immunol 1998;101(5): 672–6. Erratum in. J Allergy Clin Immunol 1998;102(1):156.

[23] Sabroe RA, Fiebiger E, Francis DM, et al. Classification of anti-FcεRI and anti-IgE auto-antibodies in chronic idiopathic urticaria and correlation with disease severity. J Allergy Clin Immunol 2002;110(3):492–9.

[24] Ferrer M, Nakazawa K, Kaplan AP. Complement dependence of histamine release in chronic urticaria. J Allergy Clin Immunol 1999;104(1):169–72 Erratum in. J Allergy Clin Immunol 2000;105(2):392.

[25] Kikuchi Y, Kaplan AP. A role for C5a in augmenting IgG-dependent histamine release from basophils in chronic urticaria. J Allergy Clin Immunol 2002;109(1):114–8.

[26] Horn MP, Pachlopnik JM, Vogel M, et al. Conditional autoimmunity mediated by human natural anti-FcεRIα autoantibodies? FASEB J 2001;15(12):2268–74.

[27] Pachlopnik JM, Horn MP, Fux M, et al. Natural anti-FcεRIα autoantibodies may interfere with diagnostic tests for autoimmune urticaria. J Autoimmun 2004;22(1):43–51.

[28] Confino-Cohen R, Aharoni D, Goldberg A, et al. Evidence for aberrant regulation of the p21Ras pathway in PBMCs of patients with chronic idiopathic urticaria. J Allergy Clin Immunol 2002;109(2):349–56.

[29] Grattan CE, Francis DM, Slater NG, et al. Plasmapheresis for severe, unremitting, chronic urticaria. Lancet 1992;339(8801):1078–80.

[30] O'Donnell BF, Barr RM, Black AK, et al. Intravenous immunoglobulin in autoimmune chronic urticaria. Br J Dermatol 1998;138(1):101–6.

[31] Grattan CE, O'Donnell BF, Francis DM, et al. Randomized double-blind study of cyclo-sporin in chronic 'idiopathic' urticaria. Br J Dermatol 2000;143(2):365–72.

[32] Gach JE, Sabroe RA, Greaves MW, et al. Methotrexate-responsive chronic idiopathic urticaria: a report of two cases. Br J Dermatol 2001;145(2):340–3.

[33] Kozel MM, Mekkes JR, Bossuyt PM, et al. The effectiveness of a history-based diagnostic approach in chronic urticaria and angioedema. Arch Dermatol 1998;134(12):1575–80.

[34] Agostoni A, Aygoren-Pursun E, Binkley KE, et al. Hereditary and acquired angioedema: problems and progress: proceedings of the third C1 esterase inhibitor deficiency workshop and beyond. J Allergy Clin Immunol 2004;114(3 Suppl):S51–131.

[35] Bork K, Fischer B, Dewald G. Recurrent episodes of skin angioedema and severe attacks of abdominal pain induced by oral contraceptives or hormone replacement therapy. Am J Med 2003;114(4):294–8.

[36] Greaves MW. Chronic urticaria as new autoimmune disease? In: Hertl M, editor. Autoim-mune diseases of the skin: pathogenesis, diagnosis, management. Wien: Springer; 2001. p. 283–302.

[37] Rumbyrt JS, Schocket AL. Chronic urticaria and thyroid disease. Immunol Allergy Clin North Am 2004;24(2):215–23.

[38] Winkelmann RK, Frigas E. Eosinophilic panniculitis: a clinicopathologic study. J Cutan Pathol 1986;13(1):1–12.

[39] Gleich GJ, Schroeter AL, Marcoux JP, et al. Episodic angioedema associated with eosino-philia. N Engl J Med 1984;310(25):1621–6.

[40] Bressler RB, Sowell K, Huston DP. Therapy of chronic idiopathic urticaria with nifedipine: demonstration of beneficial effect in a double-blinded, placebo-controlled, crossover trial. J Allergy Clin Immunol 1989;83(4):756–63.

[41] Weiner MJ. Methotrexate in corticosteroid-resistant urticaria. Ann Intern Med 1989; 110(10):848.

[42] Wong E, Eftekhari N, Greaves MW, et al. Beneficial effects of danazol on symptoms and laboratory changes in cholinergic urticaria. Br J Dermatol 1987;116(4):553–6.

[43] Parsad D, Pandhi R, Juneja A. Stanozolol in chronic urticaria: a double blind, placebo controlled trial. J Dermatol 2001;28(6):299–302.

[44] Parslew R, Pryce D, Ashworth J, et al. Warfarin treatment of chronic idiopathic urticaria and angio-oedema. Clin Exp Allergy 2000;30(8):1161–5.

[45] Wiles JC, Hansen RC, Lynch PJ. Urticarial vasculitis treated with colchicine. Arch Dermatol 1985;121(6):802–5.

[46] Nurnberg W, Grabbe J, Czarnetzki BM. Urticarial vasculitis syndrome effectively treated with dapsone and pentoxifylline. Acta Derm Venereol 1995;75(1):54–6.

[47] Jaffer AM. Sulfasalazine in the treatment of corticosteroid-dependent chronic idiopathic urticaria. J Allergy Clin Immunol 1991;88(6):964–5.

[48] Engler RJ, Squire E, Benson P. Chronic sulfasalazine therapy in the treatment of delayed pressure urticaria and angioedema. Ann Allergy Asthma Immunol 1995;74(2):155–9.

ELSEVIER
SAUNDERS

Immunol Allergy Clin N Am
26 (2006) 753–767

IMMUNOLOGY
AND ALLERGY
CLINICS
OF NORTH AMERICA

Anaphylactic and Anaphylactoid Causes of Angioedema

Paul A. Greenberger, MD

Division of Allergy-Immunology, Department of Medicine, Northwestern University Feinberg School of Medicine, 676 North St Clair Street, Suite 14018, Chicago, IL 60611, USA

Anaphylaxis was defined at a conference sponsored by the National Institute of Allergy and Infectious Diseases/Food Allergy and Anaphylaxis Network as "a severe, potentially fatal, systemic allergic reaction that occurs suddenly after contact with an allergy-causing substance" [1]. It has been described as "a serious allergic reaction that is rapid in onset and may cause death" [1]. The Joint Task Force on Practice Parameters, which represents the American Academy of Allergy, Asthma and Immunology; the American College of Allergy, Asthma and Immunology; and the Joint Council of Allergy, Asthma and Immunology, defined anaphylaxis as "a condition caused by an IgE-mediated reaction. Anaphylactoid reactions are defined as those reactions that produce the same clinical picture as anaphylaxis but are not IgE-mediated" [2]. Simons [3] has suggested that anaphylaxis be categorized as immunologic (IgE or Fc ε RI mediated), nonimmunologic, or idiopathic. Pseudoallergic is synonymous with anaphylactoid.

Incidence of urticaria and angioedema during anaphylaxis

Swelling (urticaria or angioedema) is the most common manifestation of anaphylaxis. It has been reported that urticaria likely occurs during anaphylaxis in about 90% of cases [2,3]. Angioedema appears to be much less frequent than acute urticaria when comparisons are made. For example, in a series of 91 patients referred for penicillin allergy skin testing, 52 (57%) patients had experienced urticaria and 36 (40%) patients reported non-urticarial maculopapular rash [4]. However, just 12 (13%) patients described angioedema of the tongue and face [4]. In that series, 16 (18%) patients

---

Supported by the Ernest S. Bazley Grant to Northwestern Memorial Hospital and Northwestern University.

E-mail address: p-greenberger@northwestern.edu

doi:10.1016/j.iac.2006.09.002

had at least one positive skin test reaction to the major or minor determinant penicillin skin test reagents [4]. From a series of 348 outpatients referred for skin testing, 60 (17.2%) patients similarly were positive to at least one major or minor penicillin determinant [5]. While 47 (78.3%) patients had reported having experienced urticarial lesions, 2 (3.3%) patients had developed anaphylaxis [5]. No patient had angioedema listed as the purported allergic reaction. In a series of 112 penicillin-skin-test positive patients who had experienced 143 immediate allergic reactions to penicillins, the reactions were listed as anaphylactic shock in 89 (62.2%), urticaria in 32 (22.4%), urticaria and angioedema in 21 (14.7%), and angioedema alone in 1 (0.7%) [6].

Other studies have found higher prevalence of angioedema during anaphylaxis. Angioedema was found in 40% and urticaria in 49.3% of 142 patients presenting to an ER with anaphylaxis [7]. Laryngeal edema was present in 25% of such patients [7]. In 67 patients referred to an outpatient service for evaluation of anaphylaxis, 44.8% of patients had experienced angioedema compared with 58.2% for urticaria. Dyspnea, which may have included oropharyngeal or laryngeal swelling was noted in 59.7% of patients [8]. In patients with idiopathic anaphylaxis, 335 patients, ages 5 to 83, were categorized based on whether the acute episode was generalized (urticaria or angioedema with bronchospasm, hypotension, syncope, or gastrointestinal symptoms with or without upper airway obstruction) or angioedema (urticaria or angioedema with upper airway compromise without other systemic symptoms such as shock) [9]. The patients were labeled as either IA (idiopathic anaphylaxis)-G (generalized) or IA-A (angioedema). From the 335 patients, 201 (60%) were classified as IA-G and 119 (35.5%) were designated as IA-A [9]. In this series, urticaria or angioedema occurred in all 335 patients, but anaphylaxis, implying a life-threatening emergency, involved angioedema of the upper airway in over a third of patients. Indeed, these patients had experienced laryngeal or pharyngeal edema or "massive tongue edema" [9]. Perhaps, most persuasively, in this series of 335 patients, upper airway obstruction occurred in 210 (63%) patients [9].

Angioedema in fatal cases of anaphylaxis

The importance of angioedema as a mechanism of death is highlighted from the few autopsy investigations of fatal anaphylaxis. For example, laryngeal edema was identified in 15 (37.5%) of 40 cases, but it was noted that in only 4 cases was the angioedema completely obstructing the upper airways [10]. Conversely, five of six cases reported in 1964 had pharyngeal, epiglottic, and laryngeal edema whereas the sixth patient had experienced circulatory collapse without upper airway angioedema [11]. Causes included injections of penicillin, penicillin with streptomycin, heterologous sera, bee venom, and an immunotherapy injection [11]. In a report of a fatality in a male patient with idiopathic anaphylaxis, he developed rapid onset of respiratory distress and fecal incontinence. He self-administered epinephrine. In the emergency department his blood pressure was 155/70 and pulse was 117 [12]. However, he was cyanotic and nonresponsive. "Several attempts at endotracheal intubation were unsuccessful due to edema of the hypopharynx" [12]. This finding is similar to the presence of upper respiratory tract edema in 33 (47.8%) of 69 fatal cases of Hymenoptera anaphylaxis [13]. Upper airway angioedema was present at autopsy in four (57.1%) of seven cases of food-induced anaphylaxis [14]. In a series of 56 deaths from anaphylaxis in which the death occurred within an hour in 39 cases, pharyngeal/laryngeal edema was described in 23 (41%) cases [15]. "Cutaneous erythema/urticaria" was noted in just three cases.

Most patients who experience anaphylaxis survive the episode. While acute urticaria and urticaria with angioedema occur in some 90% of cases [3], the angioedema may be of the lip or on the face or extremities instead of the pharynx, larynx, or tongue. However, the findings in fatal cases of anaphylaxis appear to be quite entirely different. Angioedema of the upper airway can be the mechanism of death, and urticaria may be infrequent. It remains unclear why when there is mast cell activation during anaphylaxis, the shock organ is the upper airway as opposed to the lower airway or vasculature. In episodes of nonfatal idiopathic anaphylaxis, urinary histamine has been found to be elevated acutely in both patients who had experienced episodes of IA-G or IA-A [16].

IgE-mediated angioedema

Penicillin

Penicillin is degraded (transformed) into the major determinate, penicilloyl-polylysine, and three minor determinants from the selections of penicillin G, sodium benzylpenicilloate, benzylpenicilloyl-n-propylamine, penicilloate, or penilloate, which can react with albumin or IgG and form immunogenic haptens. Angioedema can occur alone or as part of penicillin-induced anaphylaxis. Skin testing with the major and three minor determinants can help identify anti-penicillin IgE antibodies or, more often, exclude their presence. The positive predictive value of a history of penicillin allergy for being associated with current immunologic sensitization is approximately 11% to 18% [7,17–19] although the literature ranges from 1% to 76% [20,21]. Thus, on average, for every seven patients with a history of penicillin allergy, just one patient would be found to be skin test positive to penicillin determinants. The skin tests assist the allergist-immunologist in determining the current immunologic status in terms of administration of penicillin or other beta-lactam antibiotics. The negative predictive value of skin testing with the major and three minor determinants is from 98%

to 99% [16,18]. Seventeen percent of patients with a history of penicillin-induced urticaria or angioedema have been reported to be positive on skin testing with the major determinant, penicilloyl-polylysine and penicillin G [22]. This finding is from a study where, if a patient had experienced anaphylaxis, some 46% of patients were skin test positive compared with 7% for a history of a maculopapular rash [22].

As of October 2004, the penicilloyl-polylysine commercial product (Pre-Pen: Holister Stier, Spokane, WA) has not been made available [23]. Because from 34% to 82% of patients who are skin test positive during penicillin testing will react to penicilloyl-polylysine alone, the absence of this test reagent greatly reduces the negative predictive value of skin testing [23]. If the figure of 60% of penicillin skin test positive patients being reactive exclusively to the penicilloyl-polylysine is used, then the predictive value from negative skin tests is reduced from 99% to about 40%. Thus, the results of negative skin testing for penicillin has much less value in terms of excluding current penicillin sensitization. What if one has no penicilloyl-polylysine or minor determinants? Then, the physician is even less able to determine the immunologic sensitization at the time of the consultation. Fortunately, from 78% to 89% of patients with a history of penicillin allergy will be skin test negative to major and minor determinants, and these patients should tolerate administration of a beta lactam antibiotic without anaphylaxis. However, one would not be able to identify and presumably prevent the serious and potentially fatal anaphylactic reaction. Indeed, the previous history of anaphylaxis has been associated with as high as 46% skin test reactivity to penicilloyl-polylysine and penicillin G [22]. Cautious test-dosing can help avoid or minimize the anaphylactic reaction as compared with bolus administration [19,23,24]. Challenges should be performed when the indication is truly essential or very strongly indicated. An example of a test-dosing procedure is as follows:

1. Amoxicillin is essential or strongly indicated
2. Emergency therapy available
3. Patient exam is stable: vital signs, respiratory status, skin, (spirometry at baseline and FEV1 is at least 70%)
4. Amoxicillin (125 mg/5 mL) administered every 30 minutes if no signs/symptoms occur with final observation for 60 to 90 minutes
   a. 0.1 mL (2.5 mg)
   b. 0.5 mL (12.5 mg)
   c. 1.0 mL (25 mg)
   d. 3.4 mL (85 mg)
   e. 5.0 mL (125 mg)

A template to use during a challenge is shown in Fig. 1. For some patients, the starting dose would be lower such as with 0.1 mg followed by 1 mg, doses that would be unlikely to activate mast cells.

Medication_____

Target dose_____

Time	Dose	BP	Pulse	Skin	Chest	FEV$_1$*	Symptoms

* Respiratory status should be stable with FEV$_1$ of 70%; in occasional patients, a somewhat lower FEV$_1$ could be acceptable depending on the indication for the challenge. A physician should be present.

Fig. 1. Example of a template for a medication challenge.

Cephalosporins

Cephalosporins share the beta lactam nucleus with penicillins, yet are less likely to induce anaphylaxis [25]. There is either cross-reactivity with penicillin or independent sensitization such that penicillin-allergic patients react to cephalosporins with greater frequency than do patients who are not allergic to penicillin. Specifically, the risk of an immediate reaction with first generation cephalosporins in penicillin allergic patients has been reported to be from 5% to 16.5%, whereas for second generation cephalosporins, it is 4% (cefazolin) [23,24]. For the third and fourth generation cephalosporins, the reaction rate is 1% to 3% [23–25]. If the skin tests to the major and minor penicillin determinants are negative, cephalosporins can be administered with a great deal of safety [24,26]. However, in the absence of any skin tests for penicillin determinants, cephalosporin administration may result in anaphylaxis. Thus, the indication for the cephalosporin should be clarified, and the administration should be performed with care such as in the example in the previous section and Fig. 1. In a study of 19 penicillin allergic patients, 2 (10.5%) of 19 developed anaphylaxis from cephamandole [27]. Both patients were skin test positive to penicillin G and first received 20 mg cephamandole subcutaneously. One patient experienced "transitory hypotension, dysphonia, generalized pruritus, and upper airway breathing difficulties" [25].

The other patient tolerated the 20 mg cephamandole but next received 500 mg intramuscularly. Circulatory collapse occurred. Therefore, although most penicillin allergic patients will tolerate a cephalosporin uneventfully, and would tolerate a beta lactam antibiotic uneventfully as well, the patients who are skin test positive are at much higher risk of a severe or very severe anaphylactic reaction. Thus, caution is advised. In the absence of skin-testing reagents, the necessity of the cephalosporin should be verified. If a challenge is required, then a step-wise approach should be undertaken. The place of cephalosporin skin tests remains to be established, but experience from 101 patients is of note [28]. No patient experienced anaphylaxis if the parent cephalosporin skin test (2 mg/mL) was negative using a challenge beginning with 0.01, 0.1, and full doses. More data are needed to verify the results of negative skin testing with the parent cephalosporin.

Non-IgE–mediated angioedema

Sulfonamides

Nearly all reported allergic type reactions to sulfonamides do not mention angioedema as a primary reaction. Some evidence has been provided for the presence of antisulfamethoxazole IgE antibodies from patients who had experienced acute urticarial reactions from either sulfamethoxazole or sulfamethoxazole-trimethoprim [29]. However, because of the complexities of these investigations and the observation that most hypersensitivity to sulfonamides does not include urticaria, anaphylaxis, or angioedema, sulfonamides are presented under non-IgE mediated angioedema. Anaphylaxis has been reported in patients who have received sulfamethoxazole-trimethoprim [30,31] or trimethoprim [32]. Sulfonamide antibiotics are structurally different from nonantibiotics (furosemide, acetazolamide, celecoxib, and sulfonylureas), and the presence of a history of sulfonamide allergy does not appear to increase the risk of an allergic-type reaction from a non-antibiotic sulfonamide [23,30,31,33].

Sulfonamide therapy in patients with HIV/AIDS is associated with a greatly increased incidence of allergic-type reactions such as morbilliform rashes [23,34,35]. The administration of sulfamethoxazole-trimethoprim for *Pneumocysitis carinii* pneumonia prophylaxis and treatment is used despite highly effective antiretroviral therapy. The incidence of morbilliform rash, cytopenias, or renal or hepatic impairment ranges from 44% to 100% and typically has its onset after a week of treatment [34]. A number of potential mechanisms for allergic and idiosyncratic reactions to sulfonamides have been suggested including (1) haptenation of cell surface proteins by hydroxylamine and nitroso (oxidative) metabolites of sulfamethoxazole, (2) generation of Th1 cytokines, (3) necrotic as opposed to apoptotic cell death pathways in which necrosis causes T-cell activation and apoptosis does not, (4) reduced levels of the antioxidant, glutathione, leading to insufficient detoxification of the nitroso metabolites, and (5) slow acetylation of caffeine phenotype, which results in increased presence of the oxidative metabolites [23,34]. Alternatively, the prophylactic administration of N-acetylcysteine, which increases glutathione intracellularly, has not been shown to reduce the incidence of adverse reactions in patients [36,37]. Despite prophylactic administration of N-acetylcysteine, in the hopes of detoxifying the reactive metabolites, 20 of 96 patients receiving trimethoprim/sulfamethoxazole (80 mg/400 mg twice daily) with N-acetylcysteine (3 g twice daily) had to discontinue the antibiotics within 2 months compared with 25 of 102 patients just receiving sulfamethoxazole/trimethoprim [36]. The median time to discontinuation of the antibiotics was 13 and 14 days, and the rashes lasted about 5 days [36].

Test-dosing protocols have been suggested [24]. A history of Stevens-Johnson syndrome or toxic epidermal necrolysis is considered a contraindication to test dosing. In some cases, a report of cytopenia (or Stevens-Johnson syndrome) from a sulfonamide may have been erroneous, and a test-challenge may be indicated. Frequent evaluation and laboratory testing would be indicated to monitor the patient if there are no alternative treatments available. If a patient requires sulfamethoxazole/trimethoprim and has a history of anaphylaxis or massive angioedema attributable to sulfamethoxazole/trimethoprim, any challenge would have to be attempted after verification of the essential indication for the antibiotics. Verbal consent would be needed. The challenge would be conducted in a supervised setting with emergency therapy available as shown in Fig. 1. If there is a medical urgency, one approach would be to administer trimethoprim/sulfamethoxazole at 0.8, 7.2, 40, 80, 400, 680 mg (sulfamethoxazole) every 20 to 30 minutes [24]. Alternatively, a 4-day test-challenge would begin with 0.01 of the dose on day 1, 0.10 of the dose on day 2, 0.33 of the dose on day 3, and a full dose on day 4 [24]. Slower challenges may be indicated for some patients.

Aspirin and nonsteroidal anti-inflammatory drugs

Aspirin and non-steroidal anti-inflammatory drugs (NSAIDs) can induce acute severe bronchoconstriction (asthma), severe oropharyngeal or laryngeal angioedema, urticaria, shock, or acute nasal congestion and rhinorrhea. In a large study of patients referred for drug hypersensitivity and in which provocation challenges were performed to confirm or refute the diagnosis, 94 (47.2%) of 199 patients had a positive aspirin challenge [38]. NSAID challenges were positive in 44 (27.3%) of 161 patients [38]. Exact details of the prior or provocation-challenge reactions were not provided, but challenges consisted of aspirin at 1, 10, 20, 50, 100, 200 and 500 mg. Aspirin and NSAIDs may cause acute urticaria/angioedema in 21% to 33% of patients with chronic idiopathic urticaria [24,39,40]. Other patients will have acute urticaria/angiodema or anaphylaxis attributable to a single NSAID for example [39,41]. Convincing proof of IgE antibodies participating in such reactions has yet to be shown. Patients who experience acute urticaria or angioedema from aspirin or NSAIDs develop reactions within 3 (or possibly 4) hours in nearly all cases. Aspirin and nonselective NSAIDs inhibit cyclooxygenase-1 (and cyclooxygenase-2) enzymes which is the characteristic of the medications that induce these immediate reactions. Medications that are tolerated include cyclooxygenase-2 inhibitors (celecoxib, refecoxib, valdecoxib), and drugs that are very weak inhibitors of cyclooxygenase-1 such as acetaminophen (paracetamol), salsalate, and trisalicylate. Patients who have experienced acute urticaria or angioedema from cyclooxygenase-1 inhibitors can tolerate cyclooxygenase-2 inhibitors in almost all cases [23,24,41]. These patients can receive the first dose of the cyclooxygenase-2 either unsupervised or if there is significant anxiety, in the office. The full dose can be administered.

When aspirin or a cyclooxygenase-1 inhibitor is indicated and the patient has had a previous episode of acute urticaria or angioedema from either aspirin or a cyclooxygenase-1 inhibitor, alternative agents should be tried. However, often, the patient's disease (rheumatoid or osteoarthritis) has not responded to acetaminophen for example. With documentation that a cyclooxygenase-1 inhibitor is indicated, the patient can undergo a test-challenge with aspirin or ibuprofen (Table 1). These challenges can be performed in the office. If a patient has aspirin-exacerbated respiratory disease, it is important that the challenge be performed when the respiratory status is stable and the FEV1 is at least 70%. Use of Fig. 1 is advised. If the patient has experienced a single episode of ibuprofen-induced angioedema and if aspirin is indicated for coronary artery disease, a challenge could be performed with an initial target dose of 81 mg. It is possible that the patient has had a single episode of angioedema or anaphylaxis from another NSAID and could tolerate ibuprofen. Nevertheless, a challenge is advisable, in case the patient has class reactivity to cyclooxygenase-1 inhibitors. It is the author's opinion that the intial doses in Table 1 (aspirin 1 mg and ibuprofen 10 mg) serve as placebos. Thus, if within 5 minutes, there are symptoms or signs such as acute wheezing dyspnea, stridorous sounds, lightheadedness, or extreme anxiety, without associated evidence of airway obstruction or

Table 1
Examples of test-challenges with aspirin and ibuprofen[a]

Aspirin (dilute 81 mg tablet in water)	Ibuprofen (100 mg/5mL)
Target dose = 81 mg	Target dose = 200 mg
1 mg	10 mg (0.5 mL)
10 mg	20 mg (1.0 mL)
30 mg	40 mg (2.0 mL)
41 mg	80 mg (4.0 mL)
	50 mg (2.5 mL)

[a] The indication should be clearly documented. The patient should be observed for evidence of urticaria, angioedema, or respiratory distress. Challenges can be performed every 30 minutes in the absence of evidence of hypersensitivity.

hypotension, the patient most likely will be experiencing a panic attack and not an anaphylactoid episode. Epinephrine would not be indicated. Continued test-challenges would not be performed on that day because of the high level of anxiety. When the indication is very strong, an even faster paced challenge protocol has been described for patients with a history of aspirin or NSAID-induced urticaria or angioedema [42]. Patients were pretreated with an antihistamine (10 patients) and received a challenge as follows 0.1 mg, 0.3 mg, 1.0 mg, 3.0 mg, 10 mg, 30 mg, 40 mg, 81 mg, 162 mg, 325 mg [42]. Aspirin was administered every 10 to 30 minutes. Nine of 11 patients were able to receive aspirin without reaction [42].

Celecoxib and cyclooxygenase-2 inhibitors

The cyclooxygenase-2 inhibitors are remarkably well tolerated in patients who have aspirin-exacerbated respiratory disease (aspirin-induced asthma and aspirin triad) [24,39,41]. They also are an appropriate alternative for patients who have experienced aspirin or nonselective NSAID-induced urticaria or angioedema [23,41]. Very infrequent reports of anaphylaxis with urticaria and facial and tongue angioedema have been reported from cyclooxygenase-2 inhibitors [43]. The patient described initially had ingested a 200-mg celecoxib tablet; a repeat challenge resulted in anaphylactic shock again with a cumulative dose of 36 mg [43]. The patient subsequently tolerated rofecoxib. Thus, although rare, anaphylactic episodes can occur and physicians and their office staff should review their emergency preparedness periodically.

Acetaminophen

Extremely rare reports of acetaminophen hypersensitivity have been published [44,45]. However, acetaminophen is an appropriate alternative for aspirin or a nonselective NSAIDs for patients with aspirin or NSAID-induced urticaria or angioedema (or aspirin-exacerbated respiratory disease).

Physical urticaria

Exercise-induced anaphylaxis, a physical urticaria, is often accompanied by angioedema as well as urticaria. Exercise-induced anaphylaxis can be food-dependent and also may be associated with concurrent exposure to exercise and NSAIDs. Cold urticaria is another physical urticaria that is often accompanied by angioedema.

Immunomodulators

There are many immunomodulators, and their indications are growing. Cytokines, anti-cytokines, monoclonal antibodies, and immunosuppressive medications have provided new approaches to treatment. Adverse reactions may be profound such as the "cytokine storm" from an anti-CD28 antibody that was designed to increase the numbers of T cells and activate CD4+ CD25+ T reg cells [46]. The concentrations of tumor necrosis factor alpha (TNFα), interferon gamma (IFN-γ), interleukin (IL)-2, IL-4, IL-6, and IL-10 increased by over 2000 times in association with fever, flushing, diarrhea, hypotension, bilateral pulmonary infiltrates, and respiratory failure [46]. Aternatively, omalizumab, the anti-IgE antibody that is indicated for persistent asthma, has been associated with four immediate type reactions from more than 20,000 patients who have been treated [47]. Reactions occurred from 75 to 120 minutes after subcutaneous injection, and all patients received epinephrine. Two of the 4 patients experienced anaphylactoid reactions including one patient with throat and tongue swelling [47]. Examples of selected anaphylactic/pseudoallergic, adverse, or other immunologic reactions from immunomodulators are presented in Table 2. While there may be first-dose reactions such as the toxic "cytokine storm" from the "superagonist" anti-CD28 antibody, often there is a reaction after several uneventful administrations. This pattern suggests immunologic sensitization or idiosyncrasy.

Diagnostic contrast agents

Radiographic contrast material

Anaphylactoid reactions secondary to radiographic contrast media include angioedema, which is classified as mild laryngeal edema (moderate reaction) or severe laryngeal edema (severe reaction) [53]. Radiographic

Table 2
Examples of immunologic, anaphylactic/pseudoallergic and other reactions to immunomodulators

Therapeutic agent	Reaction
Anti-CD28 antibody	Acute respiratory failure, pulmonary infiltrates, shock; nearly fatal "cytokine storm"
Omalizumab	Anaphylaxis (75–120 minutes after subcutaneous injection) in about 1 of 5000 patients
Natalizumab	Anaphylaxis; progressive multifocal leukoencephalopathy
Infliximab, adalimumab, etanercept	Reversible SLE; anti-ds DNA antibodies
Interferon α	Acute urticaria, angioedema; anti-thyroid antibodies; SLE, diabetes mellitus, vasculitis
Rituximab, alemtuzumab	Acute urticaria, hypotension, dypspnea, rigors
Sirolimus	Angioedema; bronchiolitis obliterans organizing pneumonia; lymphocytic alveolitis
Cyclosporine	Anaphylaxis/pseudoallergic reactions
Mycophenolate	Anaphylaxis/pseudoallergic reactions
Thalidomide	Stevens-Johnson syndrome, toxic epidermal necrolysis, various rashes

Abbreviation: SLE, systemic lupus erythematosis.
Data from references [23,46–52].

contrast materials are typically tri-iodinated benzene ring compounds that are clear; thus they should not be referred to as dyes. High osmolality contrast media have osmolality from approximately 500 to 1400 mOsm/kg H_2O. Lower osmolality contrast media may have osmolality as low as 290 to 322 mOsm/kg H_2O. Lower osmolality contrast media may be nonionic or ionic. Anaphylactoid (pseudoallergic) reactions occur almost immediately to 30 minutes after intravenous administration of contrast material [53–55]. Life-threatening reactions, many of which involve cardiovascular collapse, occur within the first 20 minutes after injection of contrast media [53]. There continues to be an inadequate understanding of the pathogenesis of the anaphylactoid (pseudoallergic) reactions; there is no doubt that histamine is detected as a marker of mast cell mediator release. Various discussions of the potential pathogenic mechanisms are available [53,55]. Severe life-threatening reactions to contrast media are reduced when lower osmolality contrast materials are used compared with higher osmolality agents (0.04% versus 0.22%) [56]. Nevertheless, fatalities occur with about the same frequency (0.8 to 0.9/100,000 infusions) [57,58].

Pretreatment regimens have been published with associated low rates of repeated pseudoallergic reactions in patients who have experienced prior pseudoallergic reactions [54]. The recommended pretreatment regimen is as follows:

1. Document the essential or very strong indication for the procedure
2. Use a lower osmolality contrast medium
3. Have emergency therapy available
4. Pretreat with Prednisone 50 mg at −13 hours, −7 hours and −1 hour before the procedure
   Diphenhydramine 50 mg at −1 hour (can be oral or intravenous)
   Albuterol 4 mg at −1 hour orally is optional

With such pretreatment, only 0.5% of patients had repeated reactions. [54] There has been concern as to whether pretreatment should be recommended for patients who have had previous pseudoallergic reactions [59]. The argument appears to be based on the absence of controlled, randomized, placebo-controlled trials. Nevertheless, based on historical rates of reactions, pretreatment should be administered. Indeed, using high osmolality contrast media in patients who previously had experienced pseudoallergic reactions, the reaction rate was reduced from 17% to 60% to less than 10% with pretreatment [60]. The administration of lower osmolality contrast media to such patients reduced the repeated reaction rate to 4.0% to 5.5% and with pretreatment and use of lower osmolality contrast media, the repeat reaction rate was reduced to 0.5% [54,60].

Fatalities may occur albeit very rarely [61,62]. Thus, physicians performing such studies do need to review their emergency preparedness periodically. Pseudoallergic reactions can occur from orally administered contrast media and induce life-threatening upper airway edema [63]. Fortunately, such reactions are extremely rare.

Gadolinium

Magnetic resonance contrast media uses gadolinium-based chelates. Infrequent severe pseudoallergic reactions occur [64]. In a series of 9528 magnetic resonance imaging infusions, 45 (0.48%) patients experienced some adverse reaction. There was 1 case of anaphylactic shock (1:9528) and 15 cases of rash or urticaria. Patients who report a previous pseudoallergic reaction to gadolinium chelates appear to be at greater risk of repeated reactions [64,65]. Pretreatment of such patients and use of different gadolinium chelates are advised for essential procedures. Nevertheless, additional data are needed to confirm the efficacy of this approach.

Fluorescein

Fluorescein sodium dye is injected intravenously and can cause hypotensive shock with elevation of serum tryptase [66]. Because patients may have diabetes mellitus and coronary artery disease, an episode of shock may create a life-threatening emergency. It is not clear that any pretreatment will be successful for such patients, but this author recommends the radiographic contrast material pretreatment for such patients. The procedures should be performed only if necessary with emergency therapy available.

Summary

Anaphylactic and anaphylactoid (pseudoallergic) reactions can be expected to occur with greater frequency as the number of immunomodulators are employed. The immune system will become sensitized to these new therapeutic agents or there may be first-dose reactions depending on the pathogenetic mechanism involved. Physicians should review their office or procedure room emergency preparedness protocols and medications. The lack of penicillin major and minor determinants for penicillin testing has made management of penicillin and cephalosporin allergic patients more complicated. In the absence of skin-testing materials, test-challenges will be necessary and performed with less comfort because of not knowing the current level of immunologic sensitization to penicillin. The indication for readministration of any incriminated medication/therapeutic agent should be reviewed. Often, there are not suitable alternatives. Various approaches have been presented to permit safer readministration of essential medications or diagnostic agents to prevent episodes of anaphylaxis or upper airway angioedema.

References

[1] Sampson HA, Munoz-Furlong A, Campbell RL, et al. Second symposium on the definition and management of anaphylaxis: summary report—Second National Institute of Allergy and Infectious Disease/Food Allergy and Anaphylaxis Network symposium. J Allergy Clin Immunol 2006;117(2):391–7.

[2] Lieberman P, Kemp SF, Oppenheimer J, et al. The diagnosis and management of anaphylaxis: an updated practice parameter. J Allergy Clin Immunol 2005;115(3):S483–523.

[3] Simons FER. Anaphylaxis, killer allergy: long-term management in the community. J Allergy Clin Immunol 2006;117(2):367–77.

[4] Wong BBL, Keith PK, Waserman S. Clinical history as a predictor of penicillin skin test outcome. Ann Allergy Asthma Immunol 2006;97(2):169–74.

[5] Macy E, Richter PK, Falkoff R, et al. Skin testing with penicilloate and penilloate prepared by an improved method: amoxicillin oral challenge in patients with negative skin test responses to penicillin reagents. J Allergy Clin Immunol 1997;100(5):586–91.

[6] Romano A, Viola M, Gueant-Rodriquez R-M, et al. Imipenem in patients with immediate hypersensitivity to penicillins. N Engl J Med 2006;354(26):2835–7.

[7] Brown AFT, McKinnon D, Chu K. Emergency department anaphylaxis: a review of 142 patients in a single year. J Allergy Clin Immunol 2001;108(5):861–6.

[8] Thong BY, Cheng YK, Leong KP, et al. Anaphylaxis in adults referred to a clinical immunology/allergy center in Singapore. Singapore Med J 2005;46(10):529–34.

[9] Ditto AM, Harris KE, Krasnick J, et al. Idiopathic anaphylaxis: a series of 335 cases. Ann Allergy Asthma Immunol 1996;77(4):285–91.

[10] Delage C, Irey NS. Anaphylactic deaths: a clinicopathologic study of 43 cases. J Forensic Sci 1972;17:525–40.

[11] James LP, Austen KF. Fatal systemic anaphylaxis in man. N Engl J Med 1964;270(12): 597–603.

[12] Krasnick J, Patterson R, Meyers GL. A fatality from idiopathic anaphylaxis. Ann Allergy Asthma Immunol 1996;76(4):376–8.

[13] Barnard JH. Studies of 400 Hymenoptera sting deaths in the United States. J Allergy Clin Immunol 1973;52(5):259–64.

[14] Yunginger JW, Sweeney KG, Sturner WQ, et al. Fatal food-induced anaphylaxis. JAMA 1988;260(10):1450–2.

[15] Pumphrey RSH, Roberts ISD. Postmortem findings after fatal anaphylactic reactions. J Clin Pathol 2000;53:273–6.

[16] Greenberger PA, Miller MM. Urine histamine during episodes of anaphylaxis [abstract]. J Allergy Clin Immunol 1994;93:302.

[17] Salkind AR, Cuddy PC, Foxworth JW. Is this patient allergic to penicillin? An evidence-based analysis of the likelihood of penicillin allergy. JAMA 2001;285(19):2498–505.

[18] Warrington RJ, Simons FER, Ho WH, et al. Diagnosis of penicillin allergy by skin testing: the Manitoba experience. CMAJ 1978;118:787–91.

[19] Sogn DD, Evans R III, Shepherd GM, et al. Results of the National Institute of Allergy and Infectious Diseases collaborative clinical trial to test the predictive value of skin testing with major and minor penicillin derivatives in hospitalized adults. Arch Intern Med 1992;152:1025–32.

[20] Solensky R, Earl HS, Gruchalla RS. Penicillin allergy: prevalence of vague history in skin test-positive patients. Ann Allergy Asthma Immunol 2000;85(3):195–9.

[21] Arroliga ME, Radojicic C, Gordon SM, et al. A prospective observational study of the effect of penicillin skin testing on antibiotic use in the intensive care unit. Infect Control Hosp Epidemiol 2003;24(5):347–50.

[22] Green GR, Rosenblum AH, Sweet LC. Evaluation of penicillin hypersensitivity: value of clinical history and skin testing with penicilloyl-polylysine and penicillin G: a cooperative study of the penicillin study group of the American Academy of Allergy. J Allergy Clin Immunol 1977;60(6):339–45.

[23] Greenberger PA. Drug allergy. J Allergy Clin Immunol 2006;117(2):S464–70.

[24] Grammer LC, Greenberger PA. Drug allergy and protocols for management of drug allergies. 3rd edition. Providence (RI): Oceanside Pubs; 2003. p. 1–42.

[25] Kelkar PS, Li JT-C. Cephalosporin allergy. N Engl J Med 2001;345(11):804–9.

[26] Greenberger PA. Utility of penicillin major and minor determinants for identification of allergic reactions to cephalosporins. J Allergy Clin Immunol 2005;115(2):S182.

[27] Blanca M, Fernandez J, Miranda A, et al. Cross-reactivity between penicillins and cephalosporins: clinical and immunologic studies. J Allergy Clin Immunol 1989;83(2):381–5.

[28] Romano A, Guenant-Rodriquez R-M, Viola M, et al. Cross-reactivity and tolerability of cephalosporins in patients with immediate hypersensitivity to penicillins. Ann Intern Med 2004;141:16–22.

[29] Carrington DM, Earl HS, Sullivan TJ. Studies of human IgE to a sulfonamide determinant. J Allergy Clin Immunol 1987;79(3):442–7.

[30] Strom BL, Schinnar R, Apter AJ, et al. Absence of cross-reactivity between sulfonamide antibiotics and sulfonamide nonantibiotics. N Engl J Med 2003;349:1628–35.

[31] Hemstreet BA, Page RL. Sulfonamide allergies and outcomes related to use of potentially cross-reactive drugs in hospitalized patients. Pharmacotherapy 2006;26(4):551–7.

[32] Cabanas R, Caballero MT, Vega A, et al. Anaphylaxis to trimethoprim. J Allergy Clin Immunol 1996;97(1):137–8.

[33] Lee AG, Anderson R, Kardon RH, et al. Presumed "sulfa allergy" in patients with intracranial hypertension treated with acetazolamide or furosemide: cross-reactivity, myth or reality? Am J Ophthalmol 2004;138(1):114–8.

[34] Lin D, Tucker J, Rieder MJ. Increased adverse drug reactions to antimicrombials and anticonvulsants in patients with HIV infection. Ann Pharmacother 2006;40:1594–601.

[35] Kalanadhabhatta V, Muppidi D, Sahni H, et al. Successful oral desensitization to trimethoprim-sulfamethoxazole in acquired immune deficiency syndrome. Ann Allergy Asthma Immunol 1996;77(5):394–400.

[36] Walmsley SL, Khorasheh S, Singer J, et al. A randomized trial of N-acetylcysteine for prevention of trimethoprim-sulfamethoxazole hypersensitivity reactions in Pneumocystis carinii pneumonia prophylaxis. J Acquir Immune Defic Syndr Hum Retorvirol 1998; 19(5):498–505.

[37] Akerlund B, Tynell E, Bratt G, et al. N-acetylcysteine treatment and the risk of toxic reactions to trimethoprim-sulphamethoxazole in primary Pneumocystis carinii prophylaxis in HIV-infected patients. J Infect 1997;35(2):143–7.

[38] Messaad D, Sahla H, Benahmed S, et al. Drug provocation tests in patients with a history suggesting an immediate drug hypersensitivity reaction. Ann Intern Med 2004;140(12): 1001–4.

[39] Gollapudi RR, Teirstein PS, Stevenson DD, et al. Aspirin sensitivity: implications for patients with coronary artery disease. JAMA 2004;292(29):3017–23.

[40] Mathison DA, Lumry WR, Stevenson DD, et al. Aspirin in chronic urticaria and/or angioedema: studies of sensitivity and desensitization [abstract]. J Allergy Clin Immunol 1982;69:135.

[41] Berges-Gimeno MP, Stevenson DD. Nonsteroidal anti-inflammatory drug-induced reactions and desensitizatiion. J Asthma 2004;41(4):375–84.

[42] Wong JT, Nagy CS, Krinzman SJ, et al. Rapid oral challenge-desensitization for patients with aspirin-related urticaria-angioedema. J Allergy Clin Immunol 2000;105(5): 997–1001.

[43] Fontaine C, Bousquet PJ, Demoly P, et al. Anaphylactic shock caused by a selective allergy to celecoxib, with no allergy to rofecoxib or sulfmethoxazole. J Allergy Clin Immunol 2005; 115(3):633–4.

[44] Doan R, Greenberger PA. Nearly fatal episodes of hypotension, flushing, and dyspnea in a 47-year-old woman. Ann Allergy Asthma Immunol 1993;70(6):439–44.

[45] Vidal C, Perez-Carral C, Gonzalez-Quintela A. Paracetamol (acetaminophen) hypersensitivity. Ann Allergy Asthma Immunol 1997;79(4):320–1.

[46] Suntharalingam G, Perry MR, Ward S, et al. Cytokine storm in a phase 1 trial of the anti-CD2828 monoclonal antibody TGN1412. N Engl J Med 2006;355:1018–28.

[47] Chipps B. Systemic reaction to omalizumab. Ann Allergy Asthma Immunol 2006;97(2):267.

[48] Polman CH, O'Connor PW, Havrdova E, et al. A randomized, placebo-controlled trial of natalizumab for relapsing multiple sclerosis. N Engl J Med 2006;354(9):899–910.

[49] Champion L, Stern M, Israel-Biet D, et al. Brief communication: Sirolimus–associated pneumonitis: 24 cases in renal transplant patients. Ann Intern Med 2006;144(7):505–9.

[50] Nikas SN, Voulgari PV, Drosos AA. Urticaria and angioedema-like skin reactions in a patient treated with adalimumab. Clin Rheumatol 2006;1–2 [epub ahead of print].

[51] Krause K, Valesini G, Scrivo R, et al. Autoimmune aspects of cytokine and anticytokine therapies. Am J Med 2003;115:390–7.

[52] Stallmach A, Giese T, Schmidt C, et al. Severe anaphylactic reaction to infliximab: successful treatment with adalimumab-report of a case. Eur J Gastroenterol Hepatol 2004;16(6): 627–30.

[53] American College of Radiology Committee on Drugs and Contrast Media. Manual on contrast media, version 5.0. Reston (VA): American College of Radiology; 2004. p. 5–77.

[54] Greenberger PA, Patterson R. The prevention of immediate generalized reactions to radiocontrast media in high-risk patients. J Allergy Clin Immunol 1991;87(4):867–72.

[55] Canter LM. Anaphylactoid reactions to radiocontrast media. Allergy Asthma Proc 2005; 26(3):199–203.

[56] Katayama H, Tamagucchi K, Kozuka T, et al. Adverse reactions to ionic and nonionic contrast media. Radiology 1990;175:621–8.

[57] Caro JJ, Trindale E, McGregor M. The risk of death and of severe nonfatal reactions with high-versus-low-osmolality contrast media: a meta-analysis. AJR Am J Roentgenol 1991; 156:825–32.

[58] Cashman JD, McCredie J, Henry DA. Intravenous contrast media:Use and associated mortality. Med J Aust 1991;155:618–23.

[59] Tramer MR, von Elm E, Loubeyre P, et al. Pharmacological prevention of serious anaphylactic reactions due to iodinated contrast media: systematic review. BMJ 2006;31 [epub ahead of print].

[60] Greenberger PA. Part B: Allergic reactions to individual drugs: low molecular weight. In: Grammer LC, Greenberger PA, editors. Patterson's allergic diseases. 6th edition. Philadelphia: Lippincott, Williams & Wilkins; 2002. p. 335–59.

[61] Low I, Stables S. Anaphylactic deaths in Auckland, New Zealand: a review of coronial autopsies from 1985–2005. Pathology 2006;38(4):328–32.

[62] Wysowski DK, Nourjah P. Deaths attributed to X-ray contrast media on US death certificates. AJR Am J Roentgenol 2006;186:613–5.

[63] Seymour C, Pryor JP, Gupta R, et al. Anaphylactoid reaction to oral contrast for computed tomography. J Trauma 2004;57(5):1105–7.

[64] Li A, Wong CS, Wong MK, et al. Acute adverse reactions to magnetic resonance contrast media-gadolinium chelates. Br J Rad 2006;79(5):368–71.

[65] Nelson KL, Gifford LM, Lauber-Huber C, et al. Clinical safety of gadopentetate dimeglumine. Radiology 1995;2:439–43.

[66] Tanahasi S, Iida H, Dohi S. An anaphylactoid reaction after administration of fluorescein sodium during neurosurgery. Anesth Analg 2006;102(2):503.

ELSEVIER
SAUNDERS

Immunol Allergy Clin N Am
26 (2006) 769–781

IMMUNOLOGY
AND ALLERGY
CLINICS
OF NORTH AMERICA

Cytokine-Associated Angioedema Syndromes Including Episodic Angioedema with Eosinophilia (Gleich's Syndrome)

Aleena Banerji, MD[a], Peter F. Weller, MD[b,c], Javed Sheikh, MD[c,*]

[a]Division of Rheumatology, Allergy, and Immunology, Massachusetts General Hospital, Harvard Medical School, Cox 201, 100 Blossom Street, Boston, MA 02114, USA
[b]Division of Infectious Diseases, Beth Israel Deaconess Medical Center, Harvard Medical School, 330 Brookline Avenue, DA-617, Boston, MA 02215, USA
[c]Division of Allergy and Inflammation, Beth Israel Deaconess Medical Center, Harvard Medical School, 330 Brookline Avenue, DA-617, Boston, MA 02215, USA

Angioedema, nonpruritic and nonpitting areas of swelling in cutaneous and mucosal tissues, can involve any part of the body, but often presents as swelling of the face, lips, tongue, larynx or extremities. Angioedema may involve the gastrointestinal tract, leading to intestinal wall edema, which results in symptoms such as abdominal pain, nausea, vomiting, and diarrhea. Severe angioedema, such as acute laryngeal edema, is the major cause of angioedema-related mortality.

Angioedema, as well-considered elsewhere in this volume, can be categorized into several forms: hereditary, acquired, associated with allergic reactions (ie, venom hypersensitivity, latex allergy, adverse drug reactions, food allergy), and idiopathic. An altered production of cytokines has also been described in association with uncommon forms of angioedema. When associated with eosinophilia, the syndrome can be classified into two disorders [1,2], episodic and nonepisodic. Both of these disorders are thought to partly be caused by an alteration of cytokines. Similarly, newer monoclonal antibodies, also via cytokine alteration, have been reported to cause angioedema, although not usually associated with eosinophilia. While angioedema

---

* Corresponding author.
E-mail address: jsheikh@bidmc.harvard.edu (J. Sheikh).

0889-8561/06/$ - see front matter © 2006 Elsevier Inc. All rights reserved.
doi:10.1016/j.iac.2006.09.001 *immunology.theclinics.com*

can be caused by many factors, the authors review the literature regarding cytokine-associated angioedema syndromes.

The immune system has many different types of cells acting together to protect the human body from foreign invaders. These cells use cytokines, which are secreted proteins, to communicate. In response to an immune stimulus cytokines are produced de novo in many cells (including most types of lymphocytes), but notably exist preformed for rapid secretion in other cells, including eosinophils, basophils, and mast cells [3]. Secreted cytokines generally act over short distances and short time spans at very low concentrations. Cytokines aid cell-to-cell communication by binding to specific membrane receptors, which then signal a change in cell behavior. Responses to cytokines include increasing or decreasing expression of membrane proteins (including cytokine receptors), proliferation, and secretion of effector molecules.

The largest group of cytokines stimulate immune cell proliferation and differentiation. This group includes various interleukins, interferon (IFN)-γ, and granulocyte macrophage colony-stimulating factor (GM-CSF). Each cytokine within this group can cause a number of effects, but the major ones are as follows: interleukin (IL)-1 activates T cells; IL-2 stimulates proliferation of antigen-activated T and B cells; IL-4 and IL-5 variably stimulate T helper 2 T cells, B cells, and eosinophils; IFN-γ activates macrophages; and IL-3 and GM-CSF stimulate hematopoiesis. IL-3, IL-5, and GM-CSF are also eosinophiliopoietic cytokines.

Episodic angioedema with eosinophilia (Gleich's syndrome)

Background

Episodic angioedema with eosinophilia (EAE) was first described by Gerald Gleich and colleagues in 1984 [4]. This first report described four patients (three males, one female) with recurrent episodes of angioedema and/or urticaria, 10% to 20% increase in body weight, fever (three patients), hypereosinophilia, and an elevated IgM. Leukocyte counts were also reported to reach as high as 108,000 cells/microliter with 88% eosinophils. These four patients were followed for a period of 2 to 17 years and none of them developed organ involvement. Since 1984, many patients with similar symptoms have been reported, leading to a better understanding of this constellation of presenting signs and symptoms.

Although several hypotheses have been proposed, the exact etiology remains unclear. The main hypothesis suggests a role for helper T cells leading to an increase of cytokines including GM-CSF [5], IL-3, IL-5 [6], and IL-6 [7]. These cytokines, most specifically IL-5, are the most likely explanation for the eosinophilia observed in EAE. Others have suggested a role for anti-endothelial cell antibodies [8], vascular endothelial growth factor (VEGF) [9], IL-1, and soluble IL-2 receptor (sIL-2R) [10].

Clinical presentation and diagnosis

EAE is characterized by recurrent episodes of angioedema, urticaria, pruritus, fever, weight gain, elevated serum IgM, [6,11] oliguria, and leukocytosis with peripheral blood eosinophilia and eosinophil degranulation in the dermis. An elevated IgE has also been described [12]. Episodes usually occur every few weeks to months with complete resolution of symptoms between episodes. One patient is reported to have had remission of symptoms during an interval of 20 years before the next recurrence [4]. The level of blood eosinophilia parallels disease activity (Fig. 1). There is one case report of a woman with EAE in which her attacks were temporally related to her menstrual cycle

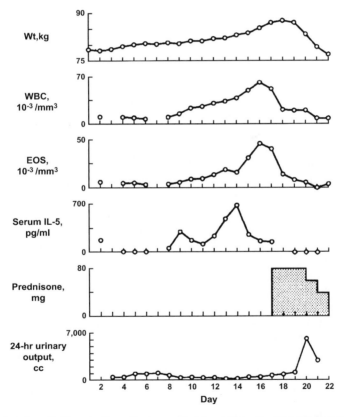

Fig. 1. Laboratory findings in the patient presented here. Note the biphasic increase in IL-5 levels. Although IL-5 levels were already decreasing on day 16, the day of maximal blood eosinophilis, predisone administration was associated with disappearance of IL-5 from the circulation. IL-5 was measured in duplicate samples of patient serum diluted 1:1 with assay diluent. The reported IL-5 value represents the mean, corrected for sample dilution. The assay detection threshold was 50 to 100 pg/mL per sample. (*From* Butterfield JH. Elevated serum levels of interleukin-5 in patients with the syndrome of episodic angioedema and eosinophilia. Blood 1992;79:689; with permission.)

[2], and another case of a young woman with EAE going through pregnancy and delivering a healthy baby despite several attacks during her pregnancy [13]. EAE has been reported in children as well as adults [14].

EAE is rare and can be difficult to diagnose, but has a good prognosis with no visceral organ involvement. EAE is now considered to be one of the several hypereosinophilic syndromes (HES) [15]. Establishing the absence of atopic, parasitic, malignant, or collagen vascular diseases is critical to making a diagnosis of EAE [15]. Awareness of this syndrome and differentiation from other forms of HES is critical because, in contrast to other forms of HES, patients with episodic angioedema with eosinophilia usually have a favorable prognosis with no organ involvement and good response to treatment [14]. The absence of cardiac damage and the episodic nature of the symptoms that correlate with eosinophil levels further distinguish these patients from those with other forms of HES [4].

Pathophysiology

The pathophysiology of this syndrome remains unclear although most researchers now agree that helper T cells and eosinophils play a central role in the disease. This is based on several studies showing an increased number of activated T cells and an elevation of specific cytokines known to activate eosinophils. In addition, high levels of eosinophils are a hallmark of this syndrome. Peripheral eosinophils can show characteristics of activation [5], although in one study they did not demonstrate the degree of hypodensity seen in hypereosinophilic syndrome patients [8].

An increased percentage of activated T cells (CD3+, HLA-DR+) was found in one report to occur 10 days before maximal eosinophilia, with no increase in activated T cells seen at the time of peak eosinophilia [6]. Some patients have clonal T-cell populations producing IL-5 [12] with peak IL-5 levels occurring several days before maximal eosinophilia [6]. Serum IL-5 levels can often become undetectable after glucocorticoid treatment [6]. IL-5 stimulates eosinophil differentiation, is an eosinophil chemoattractant and activates eosinophils; therefore, it is not surprising that IL-5 levels are elevated in EAE [6].

IL-6 is also thought to play a role, and levels have been shown to be elevated during an acute attack in one particular case [7]. IL-6 levels peaked at the same time eosinophil levels peaked and decreased as symptoms improved with the initiation of steroids. Further analysis showed an increase in IL-6 levels in blood monocyte supernatants and in skin endothelial cells, but not in blood and skin eosinophils. This suggests that elevated IL-6 levels may be due to increased production by blood monocytes and endothelial cells rather than eosinophils. The high level of circulating activated T cells [14] and cytokines suggests that EAE could be a helper T-cell– mediated disease leading to the production of various cytokines that induce inflammation and activate eosinophils. In one case of EAE, blood eosinophils were found to have upregulated C5a receptors, while neutrophils showed down-regulation of these receptors during active disease [16]. This abnormal C5a receptor expression normalized during disease remission.

Skin biopsies reveal dermal infiltration of lymphocytes and eosinophils with deposition of an eosinophil granule-derived protein, major basic protein (MBP) [14,17]. Histology shows localized, degranulated eosinophils in the dermis [4] and elevated serum levels of eosinophil major basic protein are found in these patients [17]. These data suggest that eosinophil mediators play a role in the development of cutaneous angioedema.

Lassalle and colleagues [10] describe three cases of EAE [8]. All three of these patients had anti-endothelial cell antibodies, predominantly of the IgG isotype, which were not found in controls or HES patients. Other researchers describe high basal levels of IL-1 and sIL-2R, with even higher levels of IL-1 and sIL-2R during an attack. Harada and colleagues [9] describe elevated VEGF that subsequently decreased after treatment similar to IL-5 levels in four different patients with EAE. GM-CSF has also been shown to be elevated in a patient with EAE associated with myalgias [5].

All these data, thus far, suggest that the pathophysiology of EAE is not fully understood but that is it most likely a combination of activated T cells, various cytokines, eosinophils, and possibly even immunologically induced endothelial lesions.

Treatment

Low-dose oral steroids are felt to be the best initial treatment for EAE [18]. Gleich and colleagues [4] report initially using alternate day prednisone in adults, while Morgan and colleagues [12] more recently report using 10 mg of prednisone daily with a good response. There is usually a dramatic fall in eosinophil counts to normal levels following corticosteroid therapy and symptoms of EAE resolve quickly [19]. Treatment with steroids has also been shown to induce a decrease in IL-5 and IL-6 levels [20]. The authors could find no reports of successful prophylactic treatment regimens. Patients can be asymptomatic for weeks to months or even years in between flares of EAE.

Non-episodic angioedema with eosinophilia

Background

This syndrome was first proposed by Chikama and colleagues [1] as a separate entity from EAE because it was less severe and usually limited to one attack. Non-EAE (NEAE) should be considered in patients, particularly women, who present with edema of bilateral upper or lower extremities and eosinophilia without urticaria. NEAE has been observed more frequently in Japan with almost 40 cases reported to date [21]. The cases reported in Japan seem to resolve more spontaneously than EAE and are associated with no recurrence of disease suggesting that the pathogenesis of NEAE may be different from EAE.

Clinical presentation

Shimasaki [21] describes five cases of NEAE, all in young women aged 23 to 32 years old in Japan. They all presented with angioedema, pain, and eosinophilia ranging from 4900 to 10,400/microliter. All five women are reported to have recovered spontaneously within 3 months with no recurrence of disease. These 5 cases were then compared with 25 other cases reported in Japan, looking for additional features of NEAE. There appears to be a predominance of NEAE in young females most commonly between the ages of 20 and 40 years [1,22]. There is an absence of high fevers and peripheral eosinophils are less elevated than in EAE [22]. Although IL-5 levels are elevated, they are again not as elevated as in patients with EAE. NEAE has a tendency to occur in autumn [21] and is usually one single episode of angioedema, often of the extremities. Similar to EAE, one episode can last a few months. Increased serum LDH levels have also been found [21]. These findings are consistent with the initial review in 1998 by Chikama and colleagues of 37 cases of NEAE [1]. This review suggested that IgM is not elevated in NEAE as in EAE.

Pathophysiology

The pathophysiology of NEAE is poorly understood, but as in EAE, activated T cells are believed to contribute to the pathogenesis of NEAE by recruiting eosinophils to the skin. Mizukawa and Shiohara [22] describe a marginally elevated IL-5 level (marginal in comparison to the high levels seen in EAE) and transient increase in GM-CSF during an attack, with a dramatic increase in TNF-α occurring after peak eosinophilia. This suggests that TNF-α may be involved in the resolution of symptoms (ie, eosinophil apoptosis) and plays a very different role in the pathogenesis of NEAE when compared with EAE [22]. Elevated plasma levels of the chemokine TARC/CCL17 [23] and an absence of elevated IgM [1] have been described with NEAE.

Treatment

NEAE is responsive to low-dose corticosteroid or antihistamine therapy [1,22,23], but often no treatment is needed because spontaneous remission frequently occurs [21]. This is in contrast to EAE, where spontaneous remission without any treatment is rarely seen.

Nodules, eosinophilia, rheumatism, dermatitis, and swelling

NERDS is a distinctive, relatively benign eosinophilic disorder characterized by the association of nodules, eosinophilia, rheumatism, dermatitis, and swelling [24,25]. Similar to episodic angioedema with eosinophilia, this syndrome also has a good long-term prognosis. Large, nontender compressible articular nodules arise from the tenosynovium of extensor tendons leading to episodic swelling of the hands or feet and pain in adjacent muscles and joints [24]. Biopsy of a nodule shows chronic mild tenosynovitis with numerous eosinophils and extracellular deposition of MBP [24]. Mast cells are numerous in the synovial tissue. Serum IgE values and plasma levels of eosinophil granule proteins, major basic protein (MBP), and eosinophil-derived neurotoxin (EDN) are often elevated [24].

The first patient described in the literature presented in 1967 at the age of 20 with symptoms of axillary urticaria, episcleritis, dermatographism associated with nodules, and eosinophilia. Nodule biopsy showed tenosynovitis with necrotizing granulomas, vasculitis, eosinophils, and extracellular deposition of MBP. This extracellular deposition of MBP was thought to represent eosinophil degranulation. Treatment with low-dose steroids led to disease quiescence with no symptoms for at least 15 years [24]. A second patient presented in 1990 at the age of 28 with generalized pruritic dermatitis for 15 years and eosinophilia for 2 years. This was associated with subcutaneous nodules and joint pain. Biopsy of a nodule in this patient similarly revealed mild tenosynovitis, eosinophils, and deposition of MBP. This patient is also reported to have had a relatively benign course of disease with minimal treatment. A third patient was found to have para-articular nodules, rheumatism, xerosis, recurrent urticaria with angioedema associated with tissue and peripheral blood eosinophilia [25].

These three cases show the clear association of nodules, eosinophilia, rheumatism, dermatitis and swelling leading to a diagnosis of NERDS syndrome. They all had relatively benign clinical courses. The evidence of eosinophilic involvement in these cases [24] along with the presence of activated T cells [25] suggests that cytokines are likely involved, however the details of pathogenesis of this infrequently reported disease are not known. The rarity of this condition makes it difficult to diagnose, but it is something physicians should consider in patients with idiopathic eosinophilia associated with urticaria/angioedema.

Clarkson syndrome or idiopathic capillary leak syndrome (generalized edema and monoclonal gammopathy)

Idiopathic capillary leak syndrome is a rare syndrome that was first described by Clarkson in 1960 [26]. Attacks vary in frequency, severity, and duration, but can be life threatening necessitating immediate treatment in an intensive care unit [27]. In addition to the acute form, a few cases of chronic systemic capillary leak syndrome have been described in the literature [27]. Clarkson syndrome is reported to have a 70% to 80% 5-year mortality rate [28,29] with the total duration of symptoms varying in the literature anywhere from 6 months to 7 years [30]. Thus, a broad clinical spectrum of disease has been proposed varying from episodic edema to severe hypotension, shock, and even death [27].

This syndrome usually affects individuals age 30 to 50 years with a mean age of 46 [31]. Marked thirst is described early in the attack with subsequent muscle weakness, abdominal pain, nausea, and vomiting with generalized edema. Generally, the edema appears several hours or days before the onset of acute renal failure, pulmonary edema, and shock. This is often associated with hypoalbuminemia, rhabdomyolysis, and monoclonal gammopathy. Monoclonal gammopathy, generally an IgG class, is found in more than 80% of cases. The monoclonal gammopathy needs to be closely followed since rare cases have been reported to evolve into multiple myeloma [32,33], although this remains controversial [34].

Vella and colleagues [35] describe a patient who presented with several episodes of hypotension, hemoconcentration and functional renal insufficiency. This was associated with a monoclonal gammopathy and was therefore felt to be consistent with a diagnosis of Clarkson syndrome. During the acute phase, this particular patient was treated with plasma expanders and corticosteroids. In the quiescent phase, oral aminophylline, salbutamol, and prednisone were used. After 3 months of treatment, the patient remained asymptomatic. As this case shows, early treatment with steroids during the acute phase controls many of the symptoms leading to a better prognosis [36]. In addition to plasma-expanders and steroids, terbutaline, epoprostenol, salbutamol, loop diuretics, calcium antagonists, and *Gingko biloba* extract have also been reported to show some success [27,28,30]. C1 esterase inhibitor therapy has also been reported to be successful in a small number of patients and is thought to decrease symptoms via early inactivation of the complement and contact systems [37,38]. Levels of C5a and C4d, markers of complement activation, were measured, showing normalization after C1 inhibitor treatment [37]. No prophylactic therapy has clearly proven to be efficacious although terbutaline and theophylline have shown some initial success by antagonizing vascular permeability [29,36].

The underlying cause is not fully understood, but this disorder is believed to be a result of an alteration of endothelium permeability leading to a rapid shift of plasma from the intravascular to the extravascular compartment [27]. Studies have shown IL-2 receptor–positive cells [39] and elevated soluble IL-2 receptor levels during attacks of angioedema [40] supporting the hypothesis that IL-2 causes endothelial damage leading to increased vascular permeability [27,35]. The number of mononuclear cells expressing the IL-2 receptor has been reported to be high during the capillary leakage phase [41]. Another case revealed a high C3a level suggesting that the activation of the complement pathway may play a role [31]. Adhesion molecules as well as the 5-lipoxygenase pathways have been implicated in increasing vascular permeability [36,42].

Angioedema associated with exogenous cytokine use

Aldesleukin (human recombinant IL-2)

Aldesleukin (Proleukin) is a human recombinant IL-2 product indicated for the treatment of metastatic renal cell carcinoma and metastatic melanoma and is currently under investigation for the treatment of HIV [43,44]. Aldesleukin therapy is believed to initiate a cytokine-mediated proinflammatory process resulting in a toxicity profile that is different from traditional nonbiologic chemotherapeutic agents [44]. Neutrophil activation by aldesleukin is thought to play a role in the capillary leak syndrome that can occur as a side effect of this drug.

IL-2 is a cytokine expressed by T cells that stimulates T cells, B cells, and natural killer (NK) cells and results in increased levels of IL-6, IFN-γ, and GM-CSF [44]. This leads to monocyte activation and an increase in IFN-α, IL-1, and IL-12 levels. These cytokines alter vascular permeability via neutrophils, the complement cascade, and adhesion proteins, leading to edema [44]. Aldesleukin also induces C-reactive protein, which is associated with systemic complement activation and elevated plasma levels of C3a and C5a, leading to decreased vascular integrity and further edema [44]. Aldesleukin has been associated with increased blood eosinophilia, and rarely the development of eosinophil-associated intraventricular cardiac thrombosis [45].

Additionally, there is one case report from 2003 of a patient presenting with angioedema and erythema after aldesleukin therapy. The angioedema was shown to be due to an immediate Type I hypersensitivity reaction, confirmed by enzyme-linked immunosorbent assay for specific IgE against aldesleukin, rather than cytokine alteration [43].

Angioedema with IFN-α therapy

Only a few cases of angioedema have been reported with IFN-α. In 2004, Guillot and colleagues [46] designed a prospective study to evaluate the incidence of cutaneous side effects in patients receiving adjuvant therapy with low-dose interferon for malignant melanoma. Their findings showed that almost 90% of these patients experienced one or more cutaneous side effects. The most frequent was hair loss, which occurred in 16 cases (48%). Eczematous reactions at injection sites or at remote sites were seen in 40% and pruritus occurred in 30%. In this series, one case of urticaria and one case of angioedema were reported. A second case of angioedema was reported in a patient receiving IFN-α for chronic hepatitis C infection [11]. The patient developed facial edema requiring steroids 5 months after initiation of IFN-alpha therapy, which was discontinued, and the angioedema did not recur. Other causes of angioedema including medications and hereditary/acquired angioedema were ruled out.

Table 1
Key features of cytokine-associated angioedema syndromes

Diagnosis	Angioedema	Urticaria	Eosinophilia	Ig	WBC count	Fever	Prognosis	Other features
Episodic angioedema with eosinophilia	Episodic	+/-	Yes	Increase IgM, IgE	Increase	Yes	Average	10%–20% weight gain, pruritus
Non-episodic angioedema with eosinophilia	Single episode	No	Yes	No	No	No	Good	More common in women, pain, frequent in Japan
NERDS syndrome	Episodic	+/-	Yes	IgE	No	No	Good	Nodules, rheumatism, dermatitis
Clarkson syndrome	Episodic	No	No	Monoclonal IgG	+/-	Yes	Poor	Low albumin, rhabdomyolysis and hemoconcentration

Abbreviations: Ig, immunoglubulins; NERDS, nodules, eosinophilia, rheumatism, dermatitis, and swelling; WBC, white blood cell.

Summary

Angioedema can be associated with many disorders and the presentation can be variable. Subsets of the angioedema syndromes are thought to be cytokine mediated (Table 1). Of these, the best described are the episodic angioedema with eosinophilia syndrome (Gleich's syndrome) and non-episodic angioedema with eosinophilia, which share some common features, but appear to have differences in pathophysiology. NERDS (nodules, eosinophilia, rheumatism, dermatitis and swelling), Clarkson syndrome (idiopathic capillary leak syndrome), and angioedema associated with aldesleukin (human recombinant IL-2) and IFN-α have also been reported in the literature, and have been discussed in this review. There is still much to be learned about the pathophysiology, diagnosis, and treatment of patients with these disorders. Our hope is that this review will be of help to those readers who care for patients with these disorders, and will stimulate interest in further research into the pathophysiology of these conditions.

References

[1] Chikama R, Hosokawa M, Miyazawa T, et al. Nonepisodic angioedema associated with eosinophilia: report of 4 cases and review of 33 young female patients reported in Japan. Dermatology 1998;197:321–5.

[2] Garcia-Abujeta JL, Martin-Gil D, Martin M, et al. Impaired type-1 activity and increased NK cells in Gleich's syndrome. Allergy 2001;56:1221–5.

[3] Moqbel R, Coughlin JJ. Differential secretion of cytokines. Sci STKE 2006;338:pe26.

[4] Gleich GJ, Schroeter AL, Marcoux JP, et al. Episodic angioedema associated with eosinophilia. N Engl J Med 1984;310:1621–6.

[5] Bochner BS, Friedman B, Krishnaswami G, et al. Episodic eosinophilia-myalgia-like syndrome in a patient without L-tryptophan use: association with eosinophil activation and increased serum levels of granulocyte-macrophage colony-stimulating factor. J Allergy Clin Immunol 1991;88:629–36.

[6] Butterfield JH, Leiferman KM, Abrams J, et al. Elevated serum levels of interleukin-5 in patients with the syndrome of episodic angioedema and eosinophilia. Blood 1992;79:688–92.

[7] Tillie-Leblond I, Gosset P, Janin A, et al. Increased interleukin-6 production during the acute phase of the syndrome of episodic angioedema and hypereosinophilia. Clin Exp Allergy 1998;28:491–6.

[8] Lassalle P, Gosset P, Gruart V, et al. Presence of antibodies against endothelial cells in the sera of patients with episodic angioedema and hypereosinophilia. Clin Exp Immunol 1990; 82:38–43.

[9] Harada M, Kumemura H, Yanagimoto C, et al. Vascular endothelial growth factor is involved in angioedema associated with eosinophilia. Kurume Med J 2005;52:89–91.

[10] Putterman C, Barak V, Caraco Y, et al. Episodic angioedema with eosinophilia: a case associated with T cell activation and cytokine production. Ann Allergy 1993;70:243–8.

[11] Ohmoto K, Yamamoto S. Angioedema after interferon therapy for chronic hepatitis C. Am J Gastroenterol 2001;96:1311–2.

[12] Morgan SJ, Prince HM, Westerman DA, et al. Clonal T-helper lymphocytes and elevated IL-5 levels in episodic angioedema and eosinophilia (Gleich's syndrome). Leuk Lymphoma 2003;44:1623–5.

[13] Lorraine JK. Successful pregnancy in a woman with cyclic angioedema and eosinophilia. Ann Allergy Asthma Immunol 1996;77:497–9.

[14] Katzen DR, Leiferman KM, Weller PF, et al. Hypereosinophilia and recurrent angioneurotic edema in a 2 1/2-year-old girl. Am J Dis Child 1986;140:62–4.

[15] Klion AD, Bochner BS, Gleich GJ, et al. The Hypereosinophilic Syndromes Working G: approaches to the treatment of hypereosinophilic syndromes: a workshop summary report. J Allergy Clin Immunol 2006;117:1292–302.

[16] Nakashima K, Sakurada T, Imayama S, et al. A case of episodic angioedema associated with blood eosinophilia: upregulated C5a receptor expression on eosinophils. Allergy 1998;53: 320–3.

[17] Songsiridej V, Peters MS, Dor PJ, et al. Facial edema and eosinophilia. Evidence for eosinophil degranulation. Ann Intern Med 1985;103:503–6.

[18] Emonet S, Kaya G, Hauser C. [Gleich's syndrome.] Ann Dermatol Venereol 2000;127:616–8 [in French].

[19] Schiavino D, Gentiloni N, Murzilli F, et al. Episodic angioedema with eosinophilia (Gleich syndrome). Allergol Immunopathol (Madr) 1990;18:233–6.

[20] Ray A, Sehgal PB. Cytokines and their receptors: molecular mechanism of interleukin-6 gene repression by glucocorticoids. J Am Soc Nephrol 1992;2:S214–21.

[21] Shimasaki AK. [Five cases of nonepisodic angioedema with eosinophilia.] Rinsho Ketsueki 2001;42:639–43 [in Japanese].

[22] Mizukawa Y, Shiohara T. The cytokine profile in a transient variant of angioedema with eosinophilia. Br J Dermatol 2001;144:169–74.

[23] Okamoto H, Kamatani N. Plasma concentration of TARC/CCL17 is elevated in nonepisodic angioedema associated with eosinophilia. Allergy 2005;60:1091–2.

[24] Butterfield JH, Leiferman KM, Gleich GJ. Nodules, eosinophilia, rheumatism, dermatitis and swelling (NERDS): a novel eosinophilic disorder. Clin Exp Allergy 1993;23:571–80.

[25] Zenarola P, Melillo L, Bisceglia M, et al. NERDS syndrome: an additional case report. Dermatology 1995;191:133–8.

[26] Clarkson B, Thompson D, Horwith M, et al. Cyclical edema and shock due to increased capillary permeability. Am J Med 1960;29:193–216.

[27] Airaghi L, Montori D, Santambrogio L, et al. Chronic systemic capillary leak syndrome. Report of a case and review of the literature. J Intern Med 2000;247:731–5.

[28] Fischer R, Ostendorf B, Richter J, et al. [Hypovolemic shock associated with generalized edema: paroxysmal non-hereditary angioedema (Clarkson syndrome).] Dtsch Med Wochenschr 2000;125:427–8 [in German].

[29] Tahirkheli NK, Greipp PR. Treatment of the systemic capillary leak syndrome with terbutaline and theophylline. A case series. Ann Intern Med 1999;130:905–9.

[30] Cau C. [Syndrome of increased idiopathic capillary permeability (Clarkson's syndrome).] Minerva Med 1999;90:391–6 [in Italian].

[31] Chihara R, Nakamoto H, Arima H, et al. Systemic capillary leak syndrome. Intern Med 2002;41:953–6.

[32] Amoura Z, Papo T, Ninet J, et al. Systemic capillary leak syndrome: report on 13 patients with special focus on course and treatment. Am J Med 1997;103:514–9.

[33] Hiraoka E, Matsushima Y, Inomoto-Naribayashi Y, et al. Systemic capillary leak syndrome associated with multiple myeloma of IgG kappa type. Intern Med 1995;34:1220–4.

[34] Zhang W, Ewan PW, Lachmann PJ. The paraproteins in systemic capillary leak syndrome. Clin Exp Immunol 1993;93:424–9.

[35] Vella FS, Panella E, Masciale N, et al. [Clarkson syndrome: a rare clinical condition characterized by generalized edema associated to monoclonal gammopathy.] Recenti Prog Med 2005;96:488–91 [in Italian].

[36] Garces S, Araujo F, Rego F, et al. Capillary leakage syndrome: a case report and a review. Allerg Immunol (Paris) 2002;34:361–4.

[37] Nurnberger W, Heying R, Burdach S, et al. C1 esterase inhibitor concentrate for capillary leakage syndrome following bone marrow transplantation. Ann Hematol 1997;75: 95–101.

[38] Fronhoffs S, Luyken J, Steuer K, et al. The effect of C1-esterase inhibitor in definite and suspected streptococcal toxic shock syndrome. Report of seven patients. Intensive Care Med 2000;26:1566–70.

[39] Cicardi M, Berti E, Caputo V, et al. Idiopathic capillary leak syndrome: evidence of CD8-positive lymphocytes surrounding damaged endothelial cells. J Allergy Clin Immunol 1997;99:417–9.

[40] Hoffmann U, Fontana A, Steurer J, et al. Idiopathic oedema with increased cytokine production: a pathogenetic link? J Intern Med 1998;244:179–82.

[41] Cicardi M, Gardinali M, Bisiani G, et al. The systemic capillary leak syndrome: appearance of interleukin-2-receptor-positive cells during attacks. Ann Intern Med 1990;113:475–7.

[42] Rondeau E, Sraer J, Bens M, et al. Production of 5-lipoxygenase pathway metabolites by peripheral leucocytes in capillary leak syndrome (Clarkson disease). Eur J Clin Invest 1987; 17:53–7.

[43] Abraham D, McGrath KG. Hypersensitivity to aldesleukin (interleukin-2 and proleukin) presenting as facial angioedema and erythema. Allergy Asthma Proc 2003;24:291–4.

[44] Sundin DJ, Wolin MJ. Toxicity management in patients receiving low-dose aldesleukin therapy. Ann Pharmacother 1998;32:1344–52.

[45] Junghans RP, Manning W, Safar M, et al. Biventricular cardiac thrombosis during interleukin-2 infusion. N Engl J Med 2001;344:859–60.

[46] Guillot B, Blazquez L, Bessis D, et al. A prospective study of cutaneous adverse events induced by low-dose alpha-interferon treatment for malignant melanoma. Dermatology 2004;208:49–54.

ELSEVIER
SAUNDERS

Immunol Allergy Clin N Am
26 (2006) 783–789

IMMUNOLOGY
AND ALLERGY
CLINICS
OF NORTH AMERICA

Index

Note: Page numbers of article titles are in **boldface** type.

United States Postal Service

Statement of Ownership, Management, and Circulation

1. Publication Title	2. Publication Number	3. Filing Date
Immunology and Allergy Clinics of North America	0 0 6 - 3 6 1	9/15/06

4. Issue Frequency	5. Number of Issues Published Annually	6. Annual Subscription Price
Feb, May, Aug, Nov	4	$175.00

7. Complete Mailing Address of Known Office of Publication *(Not printer) (Street, city, county, state, and ZIP+4)*

Elsevier Inc.
360 Park Avenue South
New York, NY 10010-1710

Contact Person
Sarah Carmichael
Telephone
(215) 239-3681

8. Complete Mailing Address of Headquarters or General Business Office of Publisher *(Not printer)*

Elsevier Inc., 1600 John F. Kennedy Blvd., Suite 1800, Philadelphia, PA 19103-2899

9. Full Names and Complete Mailing Addresses of Publisher, Editor, and Managing Editor *(Do not leave blank)*

Publisher *(Name and complete mailing address)*

John Schrefer, Elsevier Inc., 360 Park Avenue South, New York, NY 10010-1710

Editor *(Name and complete mailing address)*

Carla L. Holloway, Elsevier Inc., 1600 John F. Kennedy Blvd., Suite 1800, Philadelphia, PA 19103-2899

Managing Editor *(Name and complete mailing address)*

Catherine Bewick, Elsevier Inc., 1600 John F. Kennedy Blvd., Suite 1800, Philadelphia, PA 19103-2899

10. Owner *(Do not leave blank. If the publication is owned by a corporation, give the name and address of the corporation immediately followed by the names and addresses of all stockholders owning or holding 1 percent or more of the total amount of stock. If not owned by a corporation, give the names and addresses of the individual owners. If owned by a partnership or other unincorporated firm, give its name and address as well as those of each individual owner. If the publication is published by a nonprofit organization, give its name and address.)*

Full Name	Complete Mailing Address
Wholly owned subsidiary of	4520 East-West Highway
Reed/Elsevier Inc., US Holdings	Bethesda, MD 20814

11. Known Bondholders, Mortgagees, and Other Security Holders Owning or Holding 1 Percent or More of Total Amount of Bonds, Mortgages, or Other Securities. If none, check box ➤ None

Full Name	Complete Mailing Address
N/A	

12. Tax Status *(For completion by nonprofit organizations authorized to mail at nonprofit rates) (Check one)*
The purpose, function, and nonprofit status of this organization and the exempt status for federal income tax purposes:
☐ Has Not Changed During Preceding 12 Months
☐ Has Changed During Preceding 12 Months *(Publisher must submit explanation of change with this statement)*

(See Instructions on Reverse)

PS Form 3526, October 1999

13. Publication Title	14. Issue Date for Circulation Data Below
Immunology & Allergy Clinics of North America	August, 2006

15.	Extent and Nature of Circulation	Average No. Copies Each Issue During Preceding 12 Months	No. Copies of Single Issue Published Nearest to Filing Date
a.	Total Number of Copies *(Net press run)*	1,600	1,500
b. Paid and/or Requested Circulation	(1) Paid/Requested Outside-County Mail Subscriptions Stated on Form 3541. *(Include advertiser's proof and exchange copies)*	677	648
	(2) Paid In-County Subscriptions Stated on Form 3541 *(Include advertiser's proof and exchange copies)*		
	(3) Sales Through Dealers and Carriers, Street Vendors, Counter Sales, and Other Non-USPS Paid Distribution	196	211
	(4) Other Classes Mailed Through the USPS		
c.	Total Paid and/or Requested Circulation *[Sum of 15b. (1), (2), (3), and (4)]* ➤	873	859
d. Free Distribution by Mail *(Samples, complimentary, and other free)*	(1) Outside-County as Stated on Form 3541	98	98
	(2) In-County as Stated on Form 3541		
	(3) Other Classes Mailed Through the USPS		
e.	Free Distribution Outside the Mail *(Carriers or other means)*	98	98
f.	Total Free Distribution *(Sum of 15d. and 15e.)* ➤	98	98
g.	Total Distribution *(Sum of 15c. and 15f)* ➤	971	957
h.	Copies not Distributed	629	543
i.	Total *(Sum of 15g. and h.)* ➤	1,600	1,500
j.	Percent Paid and/or Requested Circulation *(15c. divided by 15g. times 100)*	89.91%	89.76%

16. Publication of Statement of Ownership
☐ Publication required. Will be printed in the November 2006 issue of this publication.   ☐ Publication not required

17. Signature and Title of Editor, Publisher, Business Manager, or Owner   Date

[signature] Jean Fanucci — Executive Director of Subscription Services   9/15/06

I certify that all information furnished on this form is true and complete. I understand that anyone who furnishes false or misleading information on this form or who omits material or information requested on the form may be subject to criminal sanctions (including fines and imprisonment) and/or civil sanctions (including civil penalties).

Instructions to Publishers

1. Complete and file one copy of this form with your postmaster annually on or before October 1. Keep a copy of the completed form for your records.
2. In cases where the stockholder or security holder is a trustee, include in items 10 and 11 the name of the person or corporation for whom the trustee is acting. Also include the names and addresses of individuals who are stockholders who own or hold 1 percent or more of the total amount of bonds, mortgages, or other securities of the publishing corporation. In item 11, if none, check the box. Use blank sheets if more space is required.
3. Be sure to furnish all circulation information called for in item 15. Free circulation must be shown in items 15d, e, and f.
4. Item 15h., Copies not Distributed, must include (1) newsstand copies originally stated on Form 3541, and returned to the publisher, (2) estimated returns from news agents, and (3), copies for office use, leftovers, spoiled, and all other copies not distributed.
5. If the publication had Periodicals authorization as a general or requester publication, this Statement of Ownership, Management, and Circulation must be published; it must be printed in any issue in October or, if the publication is not published during October, the first issue printed after October.
6. In item 16, indicate the date of the issue in which this Statement of Ownership will be published.
7. Item 17 must be signed.

Failure to file or publish a statement of ownership may lead to suspension of Periodicals authorization.

PS Form 3526, October 1999 *(Reverse)*

Moving?

Make sure your subscription moves with you!

To notify us of your new address, find your **Clinics Account Number** (located on your mailing label above your name), and contact customer service at:

E-mail: elspcs@elsevier.com

800-654-2452 (subscribers in the U.S. & Canada)
407-345-4000 (subscribers outside of the U.S. & Canada)

Fax number: 407-363-9661

Elsevier Periodicals Customer Service
6277 Sea Harbor Drive
Orlando, FL 32887-4800

*To ensure uninterrupted delivery of your subscription, please notify us at least 4 weeks in advance of move.